Physiology MCQs Made Easy

Author

DR. VARUN MALHOTRA

MD, DNB, MNAMS (Physiology), Dip. Naturopathy Yoga

Fellow of Association of Physiologists of India (ASSOPI)

Additional Professor

Department of Physiology

All India Institute of Medical Sciences

Ministry of Health and Family Welfare, Government of India

Peepee Publishers and Distributors (P) Ltd. ®

Physiology MCQs Made Easy

Published by
Pawaninder P. Vij and Anupam Vij

Peepee Publishers and Distributors (P) Ltd.
Head Office: 160, Shakti Vihar, Pitam Pura
Delhi-110 034 (India)

Correspondence Address:

7/31, First Floor, Ansari Road, Daryaganj
New Delhi-110002 (India)

Ph: 011-41512412, 011-23246245, 9811156083

e-mail: peepee160@yahoo.co.in

e-mail: peepee160@gmail.com

www.peepeepub.com

First Edition: 2024

ISBN: 978-81-9651-876-9

Dedication

In loving memory of my dear parents,

I want to take a moment to express my deep love and gratitude for the unwavering support and nurturing love you both provided throughout my life's journey. Your presence, guidance and sacrifices have shaped me into the person I am today, and I carry your teachings and values with me in every step I take.

Mom and Dad, you believed in me when I doubted myself, encouraged me when I faced challenges, and celebrated my successes as if they were your own. Your sacrifices to ensure I received a good education and your unwavering faith in my potential have been the driving force behind my accomplishments.

Though you are no longer physically with me, your love and wisdom continue to inspire me daily. This book is a testament to the values you instilled in me, the importance of knowledge you emphasized and the love you showered upon me. It is a small tribute to your memory, a reflection of the profound impact you had on my life.

I dedicate this book to both of you with all my heart, with the hope that your love and legacy will live on through these pages, reaching and touching the hearts and minds of others.

With all my love and eternal gratitude.

Varun

In profound gratitude and reverence,

I extend my deepest appreciation to my beloved Guru, Paramahansa Yogananda, and the revered Masters of India—Lord Krishna, Jesus Christ, Babaji, Swami Sri Yukteshvarji and Lahiri Mahasaya. Their divine presence and teachings have been an unwavering source of inspiration and guidance on my spiritual and yogic journey, shaping the essence of this book on **Physiology MCQs Made Easy.**

I offer this book with utmost humility, knowing that it is but a small offering in return for the immeasurable wisdom, grace and blessings I have received from each of you. May your teachings continue to illuminate the path of countless learners and bring greater awareness to the field of physiology.

With heartfelt gratitude and devotion.

Varun

Preface

The purpose of this book is to engage and educate students by presenting a comprehensive collection of multiple choice questions compiled from various postgraduate entrance exams such as AIIMS, UPSC, AP, AMC and PGI. These questions aim to challenge, evaluate and encourage students to seek additional information from standard textbooks. The emphasis is on highlighting the significance of fundamental physiology. By providing answers that reflect widely accepted views, the book intends to guide students in assuming greater responsibility for their learning. Author welcomes readers to share their suggestions, criticisms and ideas to enhance future editions.

Dr. Varun Malhotra

Acknowledgements

We express our sincere gratitude to Dr. Ajai Singh, Director of AIIMS, Bhopal, for his unwavering support in the creation of our book, **"Physiology MCQs Made Easy".** His visionary leadership and dedication to promoting Multiple Choice Questions among first-year students have been instrumental in shaping this invaluable resource. We are truly honoured to have Dr. Ajai Singh as a guiding force in our endeavour to advance the field.

Our thanks also go to Head of Department Santosh Wakode, Physiology, AIIMS, Bhopal, for his steadfast support throughout the process of bringing out this book. Dr. Wakode's invaluable guidance and mentorship have been instrumental in shaping this project, and his commitment to advancing medical education is commendable.

Special appreciation goes to my wife, Dr. Monica Malhotra, for her assistance in writing the explanations for the Respiratory System chapter.

We would also like to express gratitude to mentors, family, friends, colleagues, fellow researchers, interviewees, study participants, institutions or organizations, readers and supporters, as well as editors, publishers, illustrators, and particularly, the Peepee Publishers and Distributors (P) Ltd., for their significant contribution to the publication of **"Physiology MCQs Made Easy".**

Contents

CHAPTER 1

Central Nervous System (CNS)

What is Important in CNS?

Physiologic Anatomy of Synapse, Sensory Receptors, Motor Functions of Spinal Cord and Cord Reflexes, Functional Areas of Brain, Important Tracts

1. Which of the following reflexes disappear in the absence of functional connections between the spinal cord and the brain?

A. Swallowing reflex

B. Sweating reflex

C. Withdrawal reflex

D. Erection of penis

E. All of the above

2. What is true regarding the gamma efferent neuron?

A. A group motor neuron with a smaller diameter than that of alpha efferent neurons

B. Innervates intrafusal fibers

C. Innervates muscle fibers that stretch annulospiral endings

D. All of the above

3. Non myelinated axons differ from myelinated in that they:

A. Are most excitable

B. Lack nodes of Ranvier

C. Are not capable of regeneration

D. Are not associated with Schwann cells

4. Internuncial neurons are:

A. Essential part of withdrawal reflex

B. Essential part of stretch reflex

C. Essential part of all reflexes

D. Always excitatory

5. Aqueous humor differs from CSF in that the former:

A. Has protein content similar to plasma

B. Is an ultrafiltrate of plasma

C. Serves no important nutritive function

D. Contains a higher concentration of ascorbic acid

6. Hyperkinetic syndromes such as chorea and athetosis are usually associated with pathological changes in:

A. Motor areas of cerebral cortex

B. Anterior hypothalamus

C. Pathways for recurrent collateral inhibition in the spinal cord

D. Basal ganglia complex

7. **The cerebellum:**
   A. Has a totally inhibitory output from its cortex
   B. Has only excitatory signal output from its deep nuclear areas
   C. Has a conscious interpretation of motor activity
   D. Has inhibitory influence on muscle tone in humans

8. **A unilateral upper motor neuron lesion in the internal capsule is best characterized by:**
   A. Diminished use of contralateral appendages below the lesion
   B. Muscle fasiculations
   C. Ipsilateral hypotonicity
   D. Flexion of the leg

9. **A patient complains of muscle weakness. On administration of neostigmine, it disappears. What is its mechanism of action?**
   A. It blocks action of acetylcholine
   B. It interferes with the action of aminooxidase
   C. It interferes with the action of carbonic anhydrase
   D. It interferes with the action of acetylcholine esterase

10. **The normal amount of CSF in man is about:**
   A. 50 cc B. 100 cc
   C. 150 cc D. 200 cc

11. **A stimulus event is called a reinforcer only if it can be shown to:**
   A. Produce reduction of a homeostatic need
   B. Lead to an increased probability of response
   C. Serve as an unconditional response for operant behaviour
   D. Elicit the response that follows it
   E. Lead to generalization of response strength

12. **Increased gamma efferent discharge is seen in all except:**
   A. Anxiety
   B. Stimulation of skin
   C. Jendrassik's maneuver
   D. Rapid shallow breathing

13. **In which type of nerve fibers is conduction blocked maximally by pressure?**
   A. C B. A-alpha
   C. A-beta D. A-gamma

14. **The percentage of sensory fibers in a mixed nerve is:**
   A. 0% B. 10%
   C. 20% D. 40%

15. **Delta waves in EEG are seen in:**
   A. REM sleep
   B. Deep sleep
   C. Awake with eyes open
   D. Awake with eyes closed

16. **Satiety centre in hypothalamus is regulated by:**
   A. Gastric dilatation
   B. Blood glucose levels
   C. Blood insulin levels
   D. All of the above

17. **Upto what systolic pressure is the brain capable of autoregulation?**
   A. 65 mm Hg B. 55 mm Hg
   C. 45 mm Hg D. 75 mm Hg

18. Relation between nerve thickness and conduction velocity is:

A. Linear B. Parabolic
C. Hyperbolic D. No relation

19. Motor area of Brodman's area is:

A. 1 B. 4
C. 5 D. 7

20. CSF in comparison to blood contains all except:

A. Lower calcium B. Lower chloride
C. Lower sodium D. Lower cells

21. Vessels not under sympathetic control are:

A. Cerebral B. Splanchnic
C. Cardiac D. Cutaneous

22. The spinothalamic tract does not contain fibers for:

A. Touch sensation
B. Pressure
C. Pain
D. Discriminatory sensation

23. Resting membrane potential of nerve is equal to equilibrium potential of:

A. Na^+ B. K^+
C. Cl^- D. Ca^{++}

24. Vasomotor reflexes may be mediated through special areas of the:

A. Medulla
B. Spinal cord
C. Cerebrum
D. Hypothalamus
E. All of the above

25. First relay station of pain is:

A. Spinal cord B. Medulla
C. Pons D. Thalamus

26. A neuron which exhibits saltatory conduction differs from one which does not, in that the former:

A. Produces its action potential through potassium ion flux
B. Produces its action potential through sodium ion influx
C. Exhibits continuous conduction
D. Conducts from one node of Ranvier to the next
E. Conducts impulses more slowly

27. The speed at which an axon conducts an action potential is directly related to:

A. The diameter of dendrites
B. The diameter of axon
C. The amount of axonal branching
D. The length of axon

28. A patient with loss of function of posterior columns of spinal cord will exhibit all except:

A. Diminished vibration sense
B. Some loss of pain sensation
C. Normal plantar response
D. A clumsy gait made worse on closure of eyes

29. Muscarinic receptors are located in:

A. Membrane of effector structures innervated by postganglionic parasympathetic nerve endings
B. At neuromuscular junction on the muscle membrane
C. Membrane of parasympathetic ganglia
D. Membrane of the sympathetic ganglia

30. Cerebral cortex is generally considered to be a functional and anatomical outgrowth of:

A. Hypothalamus

B. Thalamus
C. Cerebellum
D. Midbrain

31. The EEG rhythm having lowest frequency is:

A. Alpha B. Beta
C. Delta D. Theta

32. EEG rhythm recorded from the surface of the scalp during REM sleep:

A. Alpha B. Beta
C. Delta D. Theta

33. Symptoms of cerebellar lesion include the following except:

A. Atonia B. Ataxia
C. Agnosia D. Asynergia

34. Efferent error signals from cerebellum are transmitted to the cerebral cortex via the:

A. Dentate nucleus
B. Fastigial nucleus
C. Globose nucleus
D. Emboliform

35. Normal swallowing is dependent on the:

A. Trigeminal nerve
B. Ninth and tenth nerves
C. Spinal cord
D. Pyramidal tract

36. Dorsal root fibers of spinal cord:

A. Mainly motor
B. Involved in flare phenomenon of triple response
C. Produces cutaneous vasoconstriction on stimulation
D. Involved in central control of vascular tone

37. Dreaming is usually associated with:

A. Slow waves in EEG
B. Rapid eye movements
C. Increased muscle tone
D. Decreased threshold to extrinsic stimuli

38. The alpha rhythm of EEG:

A. Has amplitude about 50 microvolts, frequency 8-12 Hz
B. Best seen when subject's eyes are closed
C. Indicates that the subject is awake
D. All of the above

39. A child demonstrates irregular spasmodic, involuntary movements of the limbs and facial muscles. He is most likely to have a lesion in the:

A. Caudate nucleus
B. Precentral gyrus of cortex
C. Post central gyrus of cortex
D. Rubrospinal tract

40. The excitatory postsynaptic potential (EPSP) differs from the end plate potential in that the EPSP is:

A. Propagated
B. A reversal of charge
C. Not associated with an increased permeability to both potassium and sodium ions
D. Not decreased by curare

41. The prime regulator of blood flow through exercising muscles is:

A. Venous tone
B. Systemic BP
C. Vasodilator metabolites
D. Sympathetic control

42. Sensory impulses originating in the periphery:

A. Ascend by unknown pathways to cortex
B. Never pass through reticular formation
C. Must all pass through reticular formation
D. Pass in part through reticular formation and in part by pass it.

43. Vomiting centre is located in:

A. Cervical spinal cord
B. Thalamus
C. Hypothalamus
D. Medulla oblongata

44. In a person with a history of alcohol abuse which of the following aspects of memory is most likely to be impaired?

A. Accurate perception of stimuli
B. Immediate recall of new information
C. Recall of events occurring a few weeks previously
D. Recognition of familiar objects

45. In cerebellar disease, all the statements are correct except:

A. The Romberg's sign is positive
B. There is Adiodokokinesia
C. There is Pendular knee jerk
D. There is involuntary tremor

46. Where is motor activity probably initiated in the brain:

A. Motor cortex
B. Premotor cortex
C. Basal ganglia
D. Cerebellum

47. The cerebellum is important in all of the following except:

A. Enabling the CNS to predict future positions of moving parts of the body
B. Initiation of muscular movements
C. Co-ordination and damping of muscular movements
D. Maintaining smooth progression of the movement

48. Almost all the cerebral cortex has direct two-way communication with which one of the following subcortical structures:

A. Cerebellum
B. Thalamus
C. Hypothalamus
D. Bulboreticular facilitatory area

49. If the connections are cut between the cortex and the thalamus, which one of the following types of brain waves can still be recorded in the cortex?

A. Alpha waves B. Beta waves
C. Theta waves D. Delta waves

50. Which of the following cortical layers is simulated most by the diffuse thalmocortical system?

A. Layer 2 B. Layer 3
C. Layer 4 D. Layer 5

51. Integration of temperature information by the nervous system occurs mainly in the:

A. Spinal cord
B. Hypothalamus
C. Amygdala
D. Peripheral receptors

52. Decerebrate animal results from the following experimental procedure:

A. Cerebrum removal
B. Transection of upper border of midbrain
C. Intercollicular transaction
D. Section above thalamus

53. Damage to which area of the cerebral cortex is likely to cause the greatest degree of loss of intellectual capabilities in a right-handed person?

A. The frontal lobes

B. The left somesthetic sensory and sensory association areas

C. The right somesthetic sensory and sensory association areas

D. The left posterior superior temporal gyrus

54. In what part of the central nervous system to the signals probably originate to provide most of the support of the body against gravity?

A. The bulboreticular facilitatory area

B. The basal ganglia

C. The motor cortex

D. The cerebellum

55. To what part of the brain do most of the signals from the Golgi tendon apparatus and muscle spindles go?

A. The somesthetic cortex

B. The thalamus

C. The basal ganglia

D. The motor cortex

E. The cerebellum

56. Hemiballismus occurring in one of the left extremities generally results from lesion in right:

A. Caudate nucleus

B. Putamen

C. Amygdaloid body

D. Subthalamic nucleus

57. The following are signs and symptoms associated with Parkinson's disease except:

A. Muscle rigidity

B. Intention tremor

C. Akinesia

D. Tremor at rest

58. The neurons in the substantia nigra which project to the globus pallidus and which are inhibitory in nature secrete at their endings:

A. Acetylcholine B. Dopamine

C. GABA D. Glycine

59. The following statements about nystagmus are true except:

A. It is present in cerebellar lesion

B. It is a symptom of vestibular lesion

C. The direction of nystagmus is in the same direction of rotation

D. Direction of nystagmus is in the same direction as that of rotation during rotation

60. Which of the following statements is not true?

A. Decorticate rigidity is greater than decerebrate rigidity

B. Righting reflexes are absent in the decerebrate animal

C. Visual righting reflex is present in a thalamic animal

D. Decorticate rigidity is seen only when the animal is at rest

61. The reticular formation is a diffuse collection of:

A. Only sensory neurons

B. Only motor neurons

C. Only autonomic centres

D. All of the above

62. Destruction of pneumotaxic centre in pons causes:

A. Apnoea

B. Forceful respiration
C. Apneustic respiration
D. Accelerated respiration

63. Bitemporal hemianopia is seen in lesions of:

A. Optic tract B. Optic chiasma
C. Optic nerve D. Occipital lobe

64. Pain carrying fibers are:

A. A α, Aβ B. A α, C
C. A δ, C D. A δ, A α

65. The fibre which is the thickest in human nerve is?

A. Touch B. Pain
C. Temperature D. Proprioception

66. True visceral pain arises from:

A. Compression
B. Irritation
C. Distention
D. Chemical stimulation

67. First neurotransmitter discovered was:

A. Dopamine B. Norepinephrine
C. 5-HT D. Acetylcholine

68. The frequency of β –waves (per sec) in EEG is:

A. 0-4 B. 4-7
C. 7-13 D. 13-30

69. Broca's area of speech lies at:

A. Superior border of frontal lobe
B. Inferior border of frontal lobe
C. Posterior border of frontal lobe
D. Superior temporal gyrus

70. Buerger waves (α- waves) of EEG have rhythm per sec as:

A. 0-4 B. 4-7
C. 8-13 D. 13-30

71. For each 1°F rise of temperature, cerebral blood flow falls by:

A. 1% B. 2%
C. 4% D. 7%

72. First synapse for peripheral sensation is:

A. Cerebellum
B. Anterior horn cells
C. Posterior horn cells
D. Midbrain

73. Wallerian degeneration of ruptured nerve starts in:

A. 6 hours B. 12 hours
C. 24 hours D. 6 weeks

74. Tremors associated with cerebellar disease are:

A. Present at rest
B. Present with action
C. Restricted to hands and trunk

75. The primary function of basal ganglia is:

A. Sensory integration
B. Short term memory
C. Preprogramming of voluntary activity
D. Control of equilibrium

76. Sensory area 1 of the cerebral cortex carries:

A. Pain fibers
B. Touch fibers
C. Fibers for fine movement
D. Tactile discrimination and two-point discrimination

77. Genu of internal capsule has:

A. Sensory fibers from thalamus to brain
B. Motor fibers from lower limb

C. Motor fibers from upper limb
D. Motor fibers from trunk

78. **Unconscious kinesthetic sensations are carried by:**
A. Anterior spinal horns
B. Spinal ganglion
C. Nucleus pulposus
D. Posterior column

79. **In a child, nerve conduction velocity reaches the adult level by:**
A. Birth B. 1-2 years
C. 3-4 years D. 6-8 years

80. **Which of the following are true of median eminence?**
A. Portion of ventral hypothalamus
B. Hypothalamus hypophyseal vessels arise here
C. Outside the blood brain barrier
D. All are correct

81. **Face is represented by.... Broadman area:**
A. I B. II
C. III D. IV

82. **The rigidity seen in Parkinson's disease is due to:**
A. Excessive stimulation of alpha motor neurons of all the muscles
B. Hypofunction of motor cortes
C. Absence of cerebellar inhibition
D. Increased sensitivity of stretch reflex

83. **The part which is electrically silent in an anesthetized preparation?**
A. Cerebellum
B. Motor area
C. Parietal area
D. Hypothalamus

84. **Right and left vagus respectively go to:**
A. SA node, AV node
B. AV node, SA node
C. AV node, bundle of His
D. SA node, bundle of His

85. **The most important factor for regulating cerebral blood flow under normal conditions is the:**
A. Rate of cerebral carbon dioxide formation
B. Rate of cerebral oxygen consumption
C. Degree of sympathetic stimulation of peripheral vasculature
D. Rate of release of potassium from the cerebrum

86. **Painful stimuli are conveyed by:**
A. A alpha and C fibers
B. B and C fibers
C. A delta and B fibers
D. A delta and C fibers

87. **The receptor protein of the muscle spindle is innervated by:**
A. Type I fiber
B. Type II fiber
C. a+b
D. None of the above

88. **The muscles typically exhibiting isometric contractions are:**
A. Extraocular B. Respiratory
C. Antigravity D. Masticatory

89. **An important facilitatory neurotransmitter mediating coitus induced ovulation is:**
A. Dopamine
B. Serotonin
C. Adrenaline
D. Noradrenaline

90. Interneurons are not functioning in .... Reflex.

A. Swallowing B. Stretch
C. Flexion D. Visual

91. No matter where a particular sensory pathway is stimulated along its course to the cortex, the conscious sensation produced is referred to the location. This is:

A. Law of projection
B. Muller's law
C. Hardy Wien's law
D. Bell Magendie's law

92. Which structures in the body are normally devoid of blood capillaries?

A. Cartilaginous plates of long bones
B. Corneas
C. Dermis of skin
D. The cartilaginous plates and the lens

93. Weber Fechner law deals with:

A. Frequency discrimination
B. Receptive field of organization
C. Intensity discrimination
D. Two point discrimination

94. Lowest level of integration of stretch reflex is at:

A. Cerebral cortex B. Upper medulla
C. Lower medulla D. Spinal cord

95. The percentage of pyramidal fibers making direct synaptic connection with motor neurons:

A. 5 B. 10
C. 30 D. 40

96. Vagotomy does not prevent the increase in gastric secretion which normally occurs in response to:

A. Injection of insulin
B. Injection of histamine
C. Sight and smell of food
D. Emotional disturbance

97. All or none law refers to:

A. Resting potential
B. Spike potential
C. Excitatory postsynaptic potentials
D. Strength of contraction

98. Bilateral lesions in lateral hypothalamic area produce:

A. Anorexia
B. Polyphagia
C. Omniphagia
D. Any of the above

99. Preganglionic sympathetic neurons stimulation causes all of the following except:

A. Secretion of saliva
B. Dilatation of pupils
C. Hepatic glycogenolysis
D. None of the above

100. The maximum rate of axonal transport is:

A. 200 mm/day B. 400 mm/day
C. 600 mm/day D. 800 mm/day

101. Renshaw cell inhibition is a typical example of:

A. Presynaptic inhibition
B. Direct inhibition
C. Recurrent inhibition
D. Recurrent excitation

102. During light sleep, the sleep spindles that appear have the frequency of:

A. 1-2/sec B. 6-12/sec
C. 14-16/sec D. 21-26/sec

103. Isometric relaxation phase lasts for ....sec.

A. 0.04 B. 0.08
C. 0.12 D. 0.14

104. The golgi tendon organ differs in function from annulospiral endings in that the tendon organ:

A. Is more sensitive to distending force
B. Causes reflex inhibition of ipsilateral heteronymous, antagonistic alpha neurons
C. Causes a reflex inhibition of homonymous alpha, efferent neurons
D. All of the above

105. What can be the most likely mechanism responsible for the abrupt cessation of skeletal muscle contraction in a normal subject attempting to lift a heavy load?

A. Activation of stretch receptors in Golgi tendon organ
B. Activation of stretch receptors in annulospiral endings
C. Skeletal muscle ischaemia
D. Inactivation of stretch receptors in Golgi tendon organ

106. The effect of sex hormones on cerebral blood flow is that it:

A. Increases
B. Decreases
C. Variable
D. None of the above

107. Extensor muscle hyperreflexia in a case of injury to midbrain between inferior and superior colliculi is due to:

A. Generalised loss of facilitation
B. Generalised loss of inhibition
C. Decreased stretch of annulospiral endings in muscle
D. Loss of inhibitions delivered to gamma efferent neurons
E. Decreased alpha efferent neuron activity

108. The following substances are not utililized or produced in fed state of brain:

A. Lactic acid
B. Pyruvic acid
C. Alpha ketoglutarate
D. All of the above

109. Which of the following may show antidromic conduction?

A. Synapse B. Axons
C. Both a+b D. None

110. Spike duration is maximum in nerve fiber:

A. A-alpha B. A-beta
C. B D. C

111. The fiber with maximum diameter is:

A. A-alpha B. A-beta
C. B D. C

112. Light reflex has its center located in:

A. Occipital cortex B. Midbrain
C. Pons D. Medulla

113. The root value of patellar reflex is:

A. L1,2,3 B. L 3,4
C. L 2,3,4 D. L3,4,5

114. Uvular reflex has afferents from cranial:

A. V B. IX
C. X D. XII

115. Sleep spindles are characterized by:

	Voltage	Frequency
A.	High	High

B. High Low
C. Low High
D. Low Low

116. All are true about brain except:
A. Energy stored
B. Can utilize fatty acids
C. Dependent on glucose
D. Sensitive to hypoxia

117. Gag reflex is mediated by cranial nerve:
A. VII B. IX
C. XI D. XII

118. Which of the following is present in high concentration in the putamen and caudate nucleus?
A. Acetylcholine B. GABA
C. Dopamine D. Histamine

119. The excitatory neurotransmitter in CNS is:
A. Serotonin B. Histamine
C. GABA D. Melatonin

120. GABA (an inhibitory neurotransmitter) acts by:
A. Increasing the permeability of a neuron to K^+
B. Increasing the permeability of a neuron to Na^+
C. Increasing the permeability to Ca^{++}
D. Decreasing the permeability of the cell to Ca^{++}

121. Chronaxie is longer in:
A. Less excitable tissue
B. More excitable tissue
C. Unexcitable tissue
D. Skeletal muscles

122. Koniocortex refers to:
A. Agranular cortex
B. Granular cortex
C. Cortex of long vertical columns
D. All of the above

123. Bathmotropic effect is produces by:
A. Stimulation of vagus
B. Nerves other than vagus
C. Atropine
D. Sectioned vagus

124. Blood brain barrier is made up of:
A. Astrocytes
B. Oligodendrocytes
C. Oligodendroglia
D. Microglia

125. The motor unit is:
A. Muscle fiber and neurons supplying it
B. Afferent fiber-centre-efferent fiber
C. Motor neuron and its muscle fibers
D. Single muscle fiber with its nerve

126. The Purkinje fibers:
A. Are myelinated axons
B. Have conduction velocity of about five times that seen in heart muscle
C. Have action potentials about a tenth as long as those in heart muscle
D. All of the above

127. Rhomberg's sign is positive in lesion of:
A. Vestibulospinal tract
B. Spinocerebellar tract
C. Spinothalamic tract
D. Any of the above

128. Golgi tendon reflex to relax muscle is:
A. Monosynaptic involving medulla

B. Monosynaptic involving spinal cord
C. Polysynaptic involving spinal cord
D. None of the above

129. CSF differs from plasma in having higher concentration of:

A. Na^+ B. K^+
C. Cl^- D. Glucose

130. Which of the following crosses the blood brain barrier most readily?

A. O_2 B. K^+
C. CO_2 D. HCO_3^-

131. Broca's area is brain area:

A. 41
B. 42
C. 44
D. None of the above

132. All of the following cross blood brain barrier readily except:

A. Water B. CO_2
C. O_2 D. Na^+

133. The band which disappears on muscle contraction is:

A. I B. H
C. A D. Z

134. Athetoid movements are found in:

A. Cerebellar lesion
B. Basal ganglia lesions
C. Thalamic lesion
D. Hypothalamic lesion

135. In spinal reflex, following are seen except:

A. Latency B. Fatiguability
C. Summation D. Memory

136. Which of the following is an example of an unmyelinated neuron?

A. Anterior horn cell
B. Preganglionic parasympathetic neuron
C. Preganglionic sympathetic neuron
D. Postganglionic sympathetic neuron

137. Which is an important reflex centre for autonomic nervous activity?

A. Cerebellum
B. Basal ganglia
C. Both cerebellum and basal ganglia
D. Hypothalamus

138. The sequence of events, i.e., Red reaction (R), flare (F) and wheal (W) in triple response is:

A. R,F,W B. R,W,F
C. W,F,R D. W,R,F

139. In brain ischaemia, systemic blood pressure rises, this is called:

A. MonroKellie doctrine
B. Cushing reflex
C. Autoregulation
D. White reaction

140. Oxygen consumption of whole human brain in ml/min is about:

A. 29 B. 35
C. 49 D. 61

141. The oxygen consumption of human brain is:

A. 1.0 ml/100 g brain/min
B. 1.5 ml/100 g brain/min
C. 3.5 ml/100 g brain/min
D. 5.0 ml/100 g brain/min

142. Pons contains:

A. Apneustic centre
B. Pneumotaxic centre
C. Carotid bodies
D. a+b

143. Which of the following factors has no direct stimulatory effect on the medullary respiratory center?

A. Changes in arterial pCO_2
B. Changes in arterial pH
C. Changes in arterial pO_2
D. Changes in the nervous output from the joint proprioceptors

144. The peripheral vasculature under the least control of sympathetic nervous system is the:

A. Artery B. Arteriole
C. Capillaries D. Venules

145. Source of EEG is:

A. End plate potential of nerve cells
B. Polarity of nerve ganglions
C. Parietal cortex
D. EPSP's and IPSP's of cortical cells which behave like dipoles

146. Transection at the level of medullary pyramids leads to:

A. Flaccidity
B. Positive grasping reflex
C. Positive Babinski's sign
D. Hypotonia

147. For arousal response, important ascending pathway is:

A. Reticulocortical
B. Corticogeniculate
C. Spinoreticular
D. Limbal

148. Blood brain barrier is maximum permeable to:

A. Na^+ B. K^+
C. Chloride D. CO_2

149. The term decerebration denotes:

A. Section of the whole cerebrum
B. Removal of one lobe of cerebral cortex
C. Removal of cerebellum from the rest of brain
D. A mid collicular section

150. Circadian rhythm is controlled by:

A. Suprachiasmatic nuclei
B. Raphe nuclei
C. Thalamus
D. Red nucleus

151. Which one of the following statements is incorrect about impulses in right auditory nerve?

A. Are initiated by distortion of hair cells in organ of corti
B. Are carried to the cochlear nuclei of medulla
C. Result in stimulation of 4th order neurons in medial geniculate body of thalamus
D. Result in stimulation of auditory area in occipital cortex

152. Superficial reflexes are:

A. Corneal B. Jaw
C. Plantar D. Both a +c

153. Principal motor area is:

A. 1 B. 2
C. 3 D. 4

154. Lowest level of integration of stretch reflex is:

A. Cerebrum B. Cerebellum
C. Pons D. Spinal cord

155. Which of the following is concerned with conditioned reflexes?

A. Cerebral cortex
B. Cerebral medulla
C. Cerebellum
D. Hypothalamus

156. Body posture and coarse movements are controlled by:

A. Cerebrum
B. Cerebellum
C. Spinal cord
D. Extrapyramidal system

157. All of the following statements about alpha rhythm of the electroencephalogram are true except:

A. It has an amplitude of about 50 microvolts
B. It has a frequency of 8-12 Hz
C. Its frequency is higher that that of the delta rhythm
D. It disappears when the subject closes his eyes

158. Anterior spinocerebellar tract ends in cerebellum through which peduncle?

A. Superior B. Middle
C. Inferior D. All

159. Match List I with List II and select the correct answer using the codes given below:

List I EEG wave	List II (Characteristic)
A. α	1. Increased when eyes are open
B. β	2. Occurs mainly in children
C. δ	3. Occurs in very deep sleep
D. Θ	4. Disappears when eyes are open

Codes

	A	B	C	D
A.	1	4	2	3
B.	4	1	2	3
C.	4	1	3	2
D.	1	4	3	2

160. Temporal lobe lesion causes:

A. Homonymous upper quadrantinopia
B. Homonymous lower quadrantinopia
C. Bitemporal hemianopia
D. Binasal hemianopia

161. The end plate potential is characterized by:

A. Propagation
B. All or none law
C. Depolarisation
D. Hyperpolarisation

162. Damage in sensory area one of the cerebral cortex results in:

A. Loss of perception of pain
B. Loss of tactile and two-point discrimination
C. Loss of perception of touch
D. Loss of only tactile discrimination

163. Excitatory synaptic transmitter substance cause which ions preferentially to move through the postsynaptic membrane?

A. Calcium B. Potassium
C. Chloride D. Sodium

164. What transmitter substance is released by the spinal nerve ending of the neurons whose cell bodies are located in the raphe magnus nucleus?

A. Endorphin B. Substance P
C. Glycine D. Serotonin

165. **All of the following manifestations are seen in cases of cerebellar damage in human beings except:**
A. Loss of non-declarative/reflexive memory
B. Loss of adjustments in vestibule-ocular reflex
C. Static tremor and rigidity
D. Ataxia, atonia and asthenia

166. **In spinal shock, reflexes are:**

	Autonomic	Somatic
A.	Normal	↑
B.	Normal	↓
C.	↑	↓
D.	↓	↑

167. **The type of nerve fiber that has a conduction velocity of approximately one metre per second:**
A. Type A alpha
B. Type A beta
C. Type A gamma
D. Type C

168. **Skeletal muscle contraction is excited when the intracellular concentration of which ion rises above 10^{11} moles per liter in the sarcoplasm of the muscle cells?**
A. Na
B. K
C. M
D. Ca

169. **Which of the following transmitter substances probably always or almost tend to inhibit the postsynaptic neuron?**
A. Gamma-aminobutyric acid (GABA)
B. Dopamine
C. Glycine
D. Norepinephrine

170. **Which sensory system might be more important for maintaining a person's balance when he is running against the wind than when he is running with the wind?**
A. Vestibular apparatus
B. Proprioceptors of the neck
C. Exterioceptive system
D. Ears

171. **Pressure on the footpads of an animal with a transected spinal cord causes the foot to:**
A. Move anteriorly
B. Move posteriorly
C. Be withdrawn
D. Thrust downward

172. **The neuronal circuit with the greatest potential for producing a long-lasting output is the:**
A. Diverging circuit with multiple inputs
B. Converging circuit with multiple outputs
C. Reverbrating circuit
D. Integrative circuit

173. **What type of neuronal circuit is typified by the nervous control of muscular activity?**
A. Diverging circuit
B. Converging circuit
C. Integrative circuit
D. Parallel circuit

174. **Match List I with List II and select the correct answer using the codes given below:**

List I (Parts of basal ganglia)	List II (Disorder)
A. Lentiform nucleus	1. Chorea

B. Subthalamic nucleus 2. Hemiballismus

C. Caudate nucleus 3. Athetosis

D. Substantia nigra 4. Parkinsonism

Codes

	A	B	C	D
A.	3	1	2	4
B.	4	1	2	3
C.	4	3	1	2
D.	3	2	1	4

175. Which theory probably explains long term memory the best?

A. The theory that it causes actual physical or chemical changes at synapses
B. The theory that there is change in RNA inside some of the neuron
C. The theory that the glial cells arouse the neuron change
D. The theory that the ionic composition of the neuron changes

176. In experimental animal, ablation of flocculonodular lobe leads to:

A. Ataxia
B. Cerebellar ataxia
C. Akinesia
D. Cerebral palsy

177. Sham rage is produced when:

A. Section is made at L2 vertebrae
B. Pons is removed
C. Medulla is removed
D. All the cortex is removed from the brain

178. Stimulation of vagus nerve causes:

A. Rise in blood pressure
B. Decreased intestinal secretion
C. Constriction of bronchial musculature
D. Relaxation of intestinal muscles

179. Osmoreceptors are present in:

A. Anterior hypothalamus
B. Internal carotid artery
C. Left atrium
D. Ventricle

180. Which one of the following pairs is not correctly matched?

Acid-base disturbance Bicarbonate, pCO_2

A. Compensated metabolic-acidosis ↓bicarbonate ↓pCO_2
B. Compensated metabolic alkalosis ↑ bicarbonate ↑ pCO_2
C. Compensated respiratory-acidosis ↑bicarbonate ↑pCO_2
D. Compensated respiratory alkalosis ↑ bicarbonate ↑ pCO_2

181. CSF pressure in the lying down posture is:

A. 20-50 mm B. 50-150 mm
C. 150-200 mm D. 200-300 mm

182. Inhibition of the spinal cord may be brought about by:

A. Glutamic acid B. Aspartic acid
C. Glycine D. Strychnine

183. When a person wishes to speak a certain thought, where does the thought originate?

A. In Broca's area
B. In the posterior part of the temporal cortex
C. In the supramarginal gyrus
D. In the facial region of the motor cortex

184. Damaging what area of the brain is likely to cause anterograde amnesia?

A. Prefrontal cortex
B. Occipital cortex
C. The amygdale
D. The hippocampus

185. Which primary cortical sensory area is located in the middle of the superior temporal gyrus?

A. Vision
B. Hearing
C. Somatic sensation
D. Taste

186. The Betz cells of the primary motor cortex is located in the middle of the superior temporal gyrus:

A. Layer I B. Layer III
C. Layer IV D. Layer V

187. Human nervous system contains about................ Neurons.

A. 10^8 B. 10^{10}
C. 10^{12} D. 10^{16}

188. Baroreceptors mainly act through:

A. Sympathetic system
B. Parasympathetic system
C. Cerebral cortex
D. Decreased blood volume

189. Parasympathetic system affects CVS mainly by altering:

A. Vascular resistance
B. Vascular compliance
C. Force of contraction of heart
D. Heart rate

190. The neuromuscular transmitter is:

A. Dopamine
B. Epinephrine
C. Norepinephrine
D. Acetylcholine

191. Destruction of lateral nucleus of hypothalamus causes:

A. Hyperphagia
B. Aphasia
C. Somnolence
D. Restlessness

192. All relay in sensory cortex except:

A. Pain B. Touch
C. Temperature D. Olfaction

193. Ultrasound refers to sound waves with a frequency of:

A. 20/sec
B. More than 20,000/sec
C. 200/sec
D. 20-200/sec

194. Nociceptive stimuli are transmitted by:

A. Free nerve ending
B. Pacinian corpuscles
C. Merkel's disc
D. Ruffini end organ

195. Cerebral blood flow begins to increase when venous blood pO_2 falls below ....mm Hg.

A. 20 B. 30
C. 35 D. 40

196. Development of myelin sheath in peripheral nervous system depends on:

A. Oligodendrocytes
B. Astrocytes
C. Microglia
D. Schwann cell

197. **Baroreceptor impulses:**
A. Inhibit the vagal centre
B. Decrease the arterial pressure
C. Result in decreased heart rate
D. Excite the vasoconstrictor centre

198. **Which of the following effects in the heart would not be a result of increased vagal nerve activity?**
A. Acetylcholine release at the nerve endings
B. Decreased ST interval
C. Bradycardia
D. Hyperpolarisation of SA node

199. **Lesions in.......lead to sensory ataxia.**
A. Posterior column
B. Vermis
C. Flocculonodular lobe
D. Vestibular apparatus

200. **EEG with spike and dome the pattern is characteristic of ....epilepsy.**
A. Jacksonian
B. Grandmal
C. Petitmal
D. Temporal lobe

201. **Sympathetic cholinergic innervation is seen in:**
A. Apocrine sweat glands
B. Eccrine sweat glands
C. Iris
D. Pancreas

202. **The existence of the "axon reflex" proves that:**
A. It has separate sensory and motor pathway inside it
B. The soma of the neuron acts as the reflex centre of the neuron
C. It can conduct impulses both orthodromically and antidromically
D. It has more than one type of neurotransmitter at its endings

203. **Bilateral destruction of auditory cortex causes:**
A. Difficulty in interpretation of sound
B. Difficulty in hearing
C. Complete loss of hearing
D. Vertigo

204. **Following percentage of pyramidal fibres make direct synaptic connections with motor neurons:**
A. 5 B. 10
C. 15 D. 20

205. **The term desynchronization indicates:**
A. S waves
B. Replacement of rhythmic with a waves
C. Replacement of rhythmic EEG pattern with low voltage, irregular waves
D. All of the above

206. **End plate potential is characterized by:**
A. Hyperpolarization
B. Normal polarity
C. Depolarization
D. None of the above

207. **At which of the following site is blood brain barrier is least effective?**
A. Cerebral cortex
B. Median eminence of hypothalamus
C. Caudate nucleus
D. Hippocampus

208. **Basic spinal postural reflex is:**
A. Flexor withdrawal reflex
B. Tonic labyrinthine reflex
C. Neck righting reflex
D. Antigravity reflex

209. The number of Na^+ channels along axons of unmyelinated neurons are:

A. 60 B. 70
C. 90 D. 110

210. Each thin filament in muscle contains ....actin molecules and.......tropomyosin molecules.

A. 100-200; 20-30
B. 200-300; 30-40
C. 300-400; 40-60
D. 800-1000; 10-20

211. The basic posture reflex is:

A. Crossed extensor reflex
B. Golgi tendon reflex
C. Flexor reflex
D. Positive supporting reflex

212. Brown Sequard syndrome, sensation lost on same side is:

A. Pain B. Temperature
C. Touch D. Proprioception

213. Which of the following is not true of the effects of trauma?

A. Hyperglycemia
B. Muscle catabolism
C. Decreased extracellular osmolarity
D. Elevation of plasma free fatty acids

214. Thirst is due to:

A. Loss of Na^+ from the interstitial compartment
B. Loss of Na^+ from extracellular compartment
C. Both
D. None

215. Posteroinferior cerebellar artery damage leads to loss of all of the following sensations except:

A. Pain B. Temperature
C. Touch D. All sensations

216. Immediately following the transaction of spinal cord in man there is:

A. A period of spinal shock that rarely lasts more than 24 hours
B. General increase in skeletal muscle tone
C. Retention of urine and feces
D. Retention of urine and feces with increase in skeletal muscle tone

217. Neurotransmitter implicated in Alzheimer's disease:

A. Acetylcholine B. GABA
C. 5HT D. NE

218. The fraction of intracellular ions normally exchanged during an action potential in unmyelinated nerve is:

A. 1/100,000 to 1/500,000
B. 1/100 to 1/500
C. 1/10 to 1/50
D. ½ to 1/5

219. pH of CSF is:

A. 7.13 B. 7.23
C. 7.33 D. 7.40

220. Which of the following has the CSF concentration more than that of plasma?

A. Glucose B. Ca^{++}
C. K^+ D. Mg^{++}

221. Which of the following has minimum CSF/Plasma?

A. Protein
B. Cholesterol
C. Uric acid
D. Lactic acid

222. Which of the following has CSF/Plasma ratio as 1.00?

A. Na^+ B. Mg^{++}
C. Cl^- D. Osmolarity

223. The value of chronaxie is minimum in:

A. Type A fibers
B. Type C fibers
C. Skeletal muscle fibers
D. Cardiac muscle fibers

224. The most ideal neurotransmitter is:

A. 5-HT
B. Substance P
C. Acetylcholine
D. All

225. On an average, the number of muscle fibers is attatched to one golgi tendon organ is:

A. 2-5 B. 5-10
C. 10-15 D. 20-30

226. The theory of membrane potential was given by:

A. Bernstein B. Nernst
C. Newton D. Foraday

227. Dysmetria is seen in:

A. Extrapyramidal lesions
B. Cerebellar lesions
C. Pyramidal lesions
D. Cortical lesions

228. Intracranial fluid in body represents:

A. 4 gm B. 100 gm
C. 40 gm D. 150 gm

229. Which is amine neurotransmitter?

A. GABA B. Epinephrine
C. Acetylcholine D. Lignocaine

230. Peripheral nerves can tolerate ischemia up to:

A. 6 hrs B. 12 hrs
C. 24 hrs D. 30 min

231. Which nerve does not have parasympathetic fibres?

A. 7 B. 9
C. 10 D. 12

232. Best method to increase, the muscle strength is:

A. Isometric exercises
B. Isotonic exercises
C. Aerobic isotonic exercises
D. Electrical stimulation

233. Autonomic ganglia are:

A. Cholinergic B. Adrenergic
C. Noradrenergic D. Dopaminergic

234. In children, cerebral flow is approximately .... that of adult.

A. Half B. Same
C. 2 times D. 3 times

235. Difference in normal resting cerebral flow in gray and white matter is ...... ml per 100 g/min.

A. 20 B. 35
C. 55 D. 75

236. Phagocytosis is done by:

A. Microglia
B. Oligodendroglia
C. Astrocytes
D. All of the above

237. Vestibular fibres relay in:

A. Vermis
B. Lateral geniculate body

C. Flocculonodular lobe of cerebellum
D. Auditory cortex

238. Most sensitive part of axon is:
A. Dendrite B. Soma
C. Axon tip D. Axon hillock

239. Most common feature of frontal lobe lesion:
A. Psychic blindness
B. Aphasia
C. Distractibility
D. Amnesia

240. The inherent rhythmicity of respiration comes from:
A. Vagus nerve
B. Pons
C. Cerebral cortex
D. Medulla

241. Striated muscle contains alternating:
A. A and Z bands
B. I and Z bands
C. A and bands
D. I and II bands

242. Which of the following parts of the cerebral hemispheres contains the auditory area?
A. Precentral gyrus
B. Postcentral gyrus
C. Superior temporal gyrus
D. Cingulate gyrus

243. In complete transaction of the spinal cord, the muscle supplied by the lower segment display:
A. Increase in tone
B. Loss of tone
C. No change of tone
D. Alternate high and low tone

244. True about nerve impulse is:
A. Travels in one direction at synapse
B. Travels in one direction along axon
C. Travels with speed of electric current
D. If current is increased too slowly, the nerve responds very fast

245. Lateral funiculus of spinal cord has all except:
A. Fasciculus gracilus and cuneatus
B. Lateral spinothalamic tract
C. Rubrospinal tract
D. Vestibulospinal tract

246. Slow muscle fibres have:
A. ↓ Endoplasmic retinaculum
B. ↓ Calcium stores
C. ↓ Glycogen
D. ↑ Mitochondria

247. Middle cerebellar peduncle transmits ....fibres.
A. Pontocerebellar
B. Tectospinal
C. Spinocerebellar
D. Olivocerebellar

248. All are synthetic senses except:
A. 2-point discrimination
B. Sterognosis
C. Vibratory sense
D. Cold sensation

249. An afferent from muscle spindles arise from:
A. The equatorial region
B. The polar region
C. Both equatorial and polar region
D. Golgi tendon organs

250. The correct sequence of parts of body represented on the motor area of cerebral cortex from above downwards is:

A. Trunk, arm, thumb, face
B. Trunk, arm, face, thumb
C. Arm, trunk, face, thumb
D. Arm, trunk, thumb, face

251. True statement regarding CSF is:

A. Daily production less than 100 ml
B. CSF analysis rules out active secretion as a mechanism of CSF formation
C. It flows from III ventricle to IV ventricle
D. Produced only by choroids plexus

252. Which of the following is mismatch?

A. Area 6: Primary gustatory cortex
B. Area 8: Conjugate movement of eyes
C. Area 24: Autonomic responses
D. Area 44: Motor area of speech

253. A positive feedback is used to our advantage in the regulation of:

A. Body temperature
B. Carbon dioxide
C. Mean arterial pressure
D. Uterine contraction during parturition

254. True about nuclear bag fibre:

A. Detects dynamic change
B. Supplied by I a sensory fibre
C. One of the type of extrafusal fibre
D. One of the type of intrafusal fibre

255. Regarding the blood brain barrier which of the following is true?

A. Prevents entry of lipid soluble substances
B. Disrupted by tumours and infections
C. Present throughout the CNS
D. All of the above

256. Thalamus is a relay station centre for all of the following sensations except:

A. Smell B. Proprioception
C. Pain D. Temperature

257. Endolymph drains into:

A. Extradural space
B. Subdural space
C. Subarachnoid space
D. Virchow Robin space

258. Precentral sulcus and corticospinal tracts are required for:

A. Voluntary movement
B. Position sense appreciation
C. Orientation in time and place
D. Stereognosis and spatial skills

259. Slow relaxation of muscle is known as:

A. Myokimia B. Myotonia
C. Myocalcemia D. Muscle spasm

260. Loss of acetylcholine receptors in the slow channel syndrome is due to accumulation of which ion in the neuromuscular junction?

A. Sodium B. Potassium
C. Calcium D. Magnesium

261. Blood brain barrier is not present in:

A. Area postrema
B. Corpus striatum
C. Corpus callosum
D. Cerebral cortex

262. The sarcotubular system is mainly concerned with:

A. Transmission of action potential
B. Muscle metabolism
C. Muscle degeneration
D. Movement of the muscle

263. Muscle is stimulated by following except:

A. α motor neuron

B. γ motor neuron

C. I α fibres

D. Type IV afferent

264. To generate the swallowing reflex integrity of chain should be upto:

A. Pyramid

B. Trigeminal nerve

C. IX and X nerve

D. Afferent central fibres to hypothalamus

265. Sweating as a result of exertion is mediated through:

A. Adrenal hormones

B. Sympathetic cholinergic

C. Sympathetic adrenergic

D. Parasympathetic cholinergic

266. Distal limb muscle tract relay through:

A. Ventral corticospinal tract

B. Lateral corticospinal tract

C. Tectospinal tract

D. Rubrothalamic tract

267. Which of the following sensations does not relay through thalamus?

A. Smell　　B. Taste

C. Touch　　D. Hearing

268. Consider the following statements. Voluntary control of respiration is:

1. Under control of cerebral cortex
2. Mediated by hypothalamus
3. The cause of exercise hyperventilation
4. Not influenced by medullary rhythmic area

Which of the following statements are correct?

A. 1 and 4　　B. 1 and 2

C. 1, 2 and 3　　D. 2, 3 and 4

269. Sympathetic stimulation causes:

A. Arteriolar constriction

B. Ciliary muscle contraction

C. Decreased gut motility

D. Decreased salivary secretion

270. The symptoms of Parkinson's disease are caused by the lesion of connection of basal ganglia at the site between:

A. Cerebral cortex and caudate nucleus

B. Putamen and substantia nigra

C. Thalamus and cerebral cortex

D. Caudate nucleus and globus pallidus

271. Match List I and List II and select the correct answer using the codes given below the lists:

List I : (Functional Division)

A. Spinocerebellum

B. Pontocerebellum

C. Vestibulocerebellum

D. Tectocerebellum

List II: (Phylogenetic Division)

1. Archicerebellum
2. Vernal neocerebellum
3. Paleocerebellum
4. Neocerebellum

Codes

	A	B	C	D
A.	3	4	2	1
B.	4	3	1	2
C.	4	3	2	1
D.	3	4	1	2

272. **Which of the following in cerebellum is excitatory?**
A. Purkinje cell B. Granule cell
C. Basket cell D. Golgi cell

273. **Reticular formation contains areas concerned with the regulation of:**
A. Hunger and thirst
B. Heart rate and hunger
C. Thirst and respiration
D. Heart rate and respiration

274. **The distance by which two touch stimuli must be separated to be perceived as two different stimuli is greater on the:**
A. Lips
B. Dorsum of hand
C. Finger tips
D. Nape of neck

275. **Repeated painful stimuli at the same site showed decrease in pain. This is caused by:**
A. Decreases in the receptive area
B. Depletion of neurotransmitter
C. Increase in threshold
D. Decrease in reflex time

276. **Afferent for segmental stretch reflex is:**
A. Secondary muscle spindle
B. Golgi tendon organ
C. 1α
D. 1β

277. **Renshaw cell inhibition is an example of:**
A. Feed forward inhibition
B. Oscillating motor activity
C. Circuitry forward
D. All of the above

278. **If one of your nerves is compressed and this leads to paresthesia for some time, the type of nerve fiber affected is probably:**
A. A α B. A αδ
C. C D. B

279. **The cortical representation for control of micturition is:**
A. Cingulate gyrus
B. Paracentral lobule
C. Frontal lobe
D. Occipital lobe

280. **Receptor which itself is a dendrite of a nerve:**
A. Olfactory B. Gustatory
C. Visual D. Hearing

281. **Which of the following is not true about action potential in skeletal muscle?**
A. Duration of action potential and muscle twitch is same
B. Action potential spreads along T tubules which releases Ca^{++}
C. Is shorter than the action potential of cardiac muscle
D. Ca^{++} in response to action potential is released from terminal cisterns

282. **When a person looks to the right side, the reflex of the impulse come from:**
A. Right motor area
B. Left motor area
C. Midbrain
D. Occiput

283. **Initiation of nerve impulse occurs at the axon hillock because:**
A. It has a lower threshold that the rest of the axon
B. It is unmyelinated

C. Neurotransmitters are release at this place
D. Most excitable and threshold high

284. Which of the following is not associated with increase in intracranial pressure?

A. Increase in blood pressure
B. Respiratory depression
C. Tachycardia
D. Deterioration of consciousness

285. Effectiveness of blood brain barrier is by:

A. Tight endothelial junction
B. Microglial cell
C. Thick basement membrane
D. Tight arrangement of astrocytes

286. All are controlled by autonomic nervous system except:

A. Aldosterone B. Insulin
C. GH D. Somatostatin

287. In brain:

A. Mesencephalic nucleus of Cr. V has multipolar neurons
B. Proprioceptive fibers of Cr. V relay in the mesencephalic nucleus
C. Fibers of the external capsule arise in frontoparietal operculum of insula
D. Fasciculus retroflexus arises from the interpeduncular nucleus

288. Complete sectioning just above the spinal cord causes:

A. Total cessation of respiration
B. Apneustic respiration
C. Cheyne Stokes respiration
D. None of the above

289. Which of the following postural reflexes is integrated in the midbrain?

A. Optical righting reflex
B. Placing reaction
C. Labyrinthine righting reflex
D. Hopping reaction

290. Auditory pathways pass through all of the following structures except:

A. Coclear nuclei
B. Superior olives
C. Trapezoid body
D. Superior colliculus

291. Pyrogens raise body temperature by:

A. Setting the thermostat to higher level
B. Releasing interleukins
C. Decreasing peripheral heat liberating mechanism
D. Causing peripheral vasoconstriction

292. The cells of cochlea are called as:

A. Etitheliophorial
B. Outer and Inner hair cells
C. Transitional apical hair cells
D. None of these

293. Which type of cell in the visual cortex responds best to a moving bar of light?

A. Simple B. Complex
C. Hypercomplex D. Bipolar

294. Climbing fibres are:

A. Output fibre
B. Excitatory fibre
C. Comes from superior olivary nucleus
D. Comes from multiple source

295. Lesion in Inferior frontal gyri shows:

A. Difficulty in articulation
B. Compromised language output

C. Inability to comprehend written language

D. Inability to comprehend hearing

296. True about alpha block is all except:

A. Low irregular voltage

B. Mental alertness

C. Desynchronisation

D. Synchronisation

297. A dog was fed always while ringing a bell, then whenever the bell was rung it salivated here the bell acts as a:

A. Reinforcer B. Conditioner

C. Non-conditioner D. Facilitater

298. Which of the following is true about autonomic nervous system?

A. The sympathetic outflow from the CNS is through both the cranial nerves and sympathetic chain

B. The parasympathetic outflow from the CNS is through the cranial nerves only

C. The superior hypogastric plexus is located at the anterior aspect of the aortic bifurcation and the fifth lumbar vertebrae

D. The superior hypogastric plexus contains sympathetic chain

299. Synaptic conduction is mostly orthodromic because:

A. Dendrites cannot be repolarised

B. Once repolarised, an area cannot be repolarised

C. The strength of antidromic impulse is less

D. Chemical mediator is located only in the presynaptic terminal

EXPLANATORY ANSWERS OF CNS

1. **Ans. A:** Swallowing reflex is a brainstem reflex. The others are local spinal reflexes that will be intact even when the higher centres in the brain are severed from the lower centres. (AK Jain 213, 214)

2. **Ans. D:** Gamma motor neuron helps to passively and actively stretch the muscle spindle in readiness for the muscle to contract. (AK Jain 900, 903)

3. **Ans. B:** Nonmyelinated axons are present in the brain, as myelination sheath cannot be accommodated in the small space of the brain. Myelinated axons conduct faster, saltatory conduction (jumping of a frog), from one node of Ranvier to the other. (AK Jain 142, 148)

4. **Ans. A:** Internuncial neurons are located in the spinal cord. They play a role in the withdrawal reflex in response to pain. It is a protective response, involving activation of neurons on both sides of the body. (AK Jain 906, 907)

5. **Ans. D:** Aqueous humor, present in the anterior chamber of the eye provides nutrition to the lens and structures present therein. It is drained by the canal of Schlemm. (AK Jain 1121, 1122)

6. **Ans. D:** Athetosis is slow writhing snake like movements seen in lesion of lentiform nucleus. Chorea is fast, dancing like movement due to lesions of caudate nucleus of the basal ganglia. Hemiballismus are violent movements of half side of the body. All are involuntary in nature. They may be controlled by Dopamine agonists. (AK Jain 1030)

7. **Ans. A:** Cerebellar lesions produce hypotonia in humans. It compares the motor plan from basal ganglia and proprioceptive, exterioceptive inputs from joints and five senses with the desired goal oriented action signal from the cortex. It corrects the discrepancy between the two to smoothen the motion in rate, range and force. (AK Jain 998)

8. **Ans. A:** Contralateral hemiplegia occurs commonly here in ischemia of the lenticulo-striate artery supplying the pyramidal motor tract. (AK Jain 940, 942)

9. **Ans. D:** Neostigmine is the drug of choice for Myasthenia gravis. It interferes with the action of acetylcholine esterase, to increase the concentration of acetylcholine in the synaptic cleft, to produce an increase in MEPP (Miniature End Plate Potential). (AK Jain 160, 778)

10. **Ans. C:** Decrease in volume of CSF results in headache especially seen as a complication after lumbar puncture. (AK Jain 389-393)

11. **Ans. B:** Reinforcement and repetition activate the reverberatory Papez circuits to form neural proteins in development of long-term memory (LTP: Long term potentiation). (AK Jain 2, 1071)

12. **Ans. D:** Rapid deep breathing, and conditions increasing the supraspinal influences (Gamma motor neuron discharge) produce an alert, aroused state, preparing the person for action. (AK Jain 900, 903).

13. **Ans. C:** A fiber is most susceptible to pressure. Aβ conducts touch and pressure. (AK Jain 149, 150)

14. **Ans. D:** Sensory fibers conduct electrical impulses from the periphery to the brain.

Motor nerves conduct electrical impulses from the brain to the periphery. (AK Jain 975)

15. **Ans. B:** Pontogeniculate occipital spikes are seen in REM sleep. Alpha rhythm is seen in awake with eyes closed, showing a relaxed but aware state. Beta rhythm or desynchronized rhythm is seen when awake with eyes open showing an alert and aroused state. (AK Jain 1017)

16. **Ans. B:** The ventromedial nucleus or satiety centre is the only part of the brain that requires insulin for utilization of blood glucose. The difference between arteriovenous levels of glucose regulate the activity of the ventromedial nucleus. (AK Jain 1037)

17. **Ans. A:** Last ditch response or CNS ischemic response to increase blood pressure operates at the level of medulla to cause intense vasoconstriction and increase in sympathetic drive. (AK Jain 367)

18. **Ans. A:** Thicker the nerve cables, faster the flow of electrons (current). Proprioceptive impulses from the joint are thick cables relaying information to the brain about body position. (AK Jain 149,150)

19. **Ans. B:** Ischemia in Brodmann's area 4 leads to monoplegia (paralysis of one limb). (AK Jain 940)

20. **Ans. B:** CSF tap yield is sent to microbiology for culture, pathology for cells and biochemistry for estimation of blood glucose. A traumatic tap can be differentiated from a subarachnoid haemorrhage in that the change of colour of CSF from reddish to colourless in the former, as blood clots. In the latter the red CSF colour persists in all three vials. (AK Jain 389-393)

21. **Ans. A:** During exercise redistribution of blood flow occurs to the heart and working muscles from the splanchnic bed and skin. The blood to the brain is kept constant. (AK Jain 505)

22. **Ans. D:** PSVT: Proprioception, Somatic localization and discrimination, vibration and touch are carried by the dorsal column. (AK Jain 914, 916)

23. **Ans. C:** At -70 mv the resting membrane potential, chloride ions freely diffuse into and out of the cell, as it is in electrochemical equilibrium to this potential. (AK Jain 32, 36)

24. **Ans. E:** The medulla the integrator of baroreceptor, chemoreceptor vasomotor reflexes. Spinal cord the site of axon reflex and many locally mediated reflexes. Cerebrum the initiator of cortico-hypothalamic descending pathway. Hypothalamus is the head ganglion of the autonomic nervous system (Sherrington). (AK Jain 342, 414)

25. **Ans. A:** Gate control theory of pain has its relay site at the rexed laminae of the spinal cord. A δ and C fibers relay to the spinal cord fast and slow pain. They are sharp in nature, from periphery and dull from the viscera, respectively. (AK Jain 927-928)

26. **Ans. D:** Myelinated axons conduct faster, saltatory conduction (jumping of a frog), from one node of Ranvier to the other. (AK Jain 142,148)

27. **Ans. B:** Thicker the nerve cables, faster the flow of electrons (current). Proprioceptive impulses from the joint are thick cables relaying information to the brain about body position. (AK Jain 149,150)

28. **Ans. B:** Choice D is Rhomberg's sign or sensory ataxia seen in Tabes dorsalis

and conditions affecting posterior column. Pain is carried by the lateral spinothalamic tract. Proprioception, Somatic localization, vibration and touch are carried by the dorsal column. (AK Jain 914, 915)

29. **Ans. A:** Muscarinic receptors M_3 are present in the parietal cell. Nicotinic receptors are located in the motor end plate. (A K Jain 158)

30. **Ans. B:** Thalamus is a subcortical group of nuclei that forms a relay station for sensory stimuli, in humans after encephalization took place. In birds the thalamus forms a higher cortical structure. (AK Jain 1009)

31. **Ans. D:** Frequency of alpha wave is 8-12 Hz, beta waves is 14-30 Hz, Theta 4-7 z, Delta 1-4 Hz. (AK Jain 1012)

32. **Ans. A:** REM sleep produces PGO spikes which are present in the occipital and parietal region. These are alpha like waves. (AK Jain 1018)

33. **Ans. C:** Ataxia is incoordination of movement marked by asynergia–lack of coordination between antagonists and synergists. Dysmetria is movement that is poorly carried out in direction, range and force. (A K Jain 1002)

34. **Ans. A:** The cerebral-cerebellar-cerebral circuit is *cortico-ponto-dentato-thalamo-cortical circuit.* It compares the motor plan from basal ganglia and propioceptive, exterioceptive inputs from joints and five senses with the desired goal oriented action signal from the cortex. It corrects the discrepancy between the two to smoothen the motion in rate, range and force. (AK Jain 998)

35. **Ans. B:** Gag reflex involves afferent as IX nerve and efferent as vagus nerve. Deglutition apnea also involves these nerves. (AK Jain 873)

36. **Ans. B:** Axon reflex or Triple response is redness, wheal and flare (spread of the redness). The neurotransmitters involved are histamine, CGRP, Substance P. (A K Jain 341)

37. **Ans. B:** Dreaming occurs in REM sleep and Non dreaming sleep in NREM sleep.

38. **Ans. D:** Alpha rhythm reflects aware, but relaxed state, as eyes are closed. (AK Jain 1012)

39. **Ans. A:** This is a manifestation of chorea. Chorea is fast, dancing like movement due to lesions of caudate nucleus of the basal ganglia. (AK Jain 1030)

40. **Ans. D:** d-tubocurarine competes with aceylcholine to decrease end plate potential. (AK Jain 952, 158)

41. **Ans. C:** Hypoxia and increase in carbon dioxide accumulation causes vasodilation, that causes redistribution of blood flow to the active muscles during exercise. (AK Jain 505)

42. **Ans. D:** Pass in part through reticular formation (non specific relay system) and in part bypass it (specific ascending pathway). They form multisynaptic relays to widespread areas of the cortex. The specific pathway forms rapid relay to the cortex. (Ganong 195)

43. **Ans. D:** Vomiting centre is associated with chemoreceptor zone (CTZ) of area postrema in the medulla. Apomorphine, copper sulphate may be used to induce vomiting in cases of poisoning. Other emetic agents include digitalis and glycosides. (Ganong 236)

44. **Ans. C:** Korsakoff's syndrome due to alcohol abuse involves the hippocampus and involves retrograde amnesia, loss of recent memory. (Ganong 274)

45. **Ans. D:** Tremor of cerebellar disease appears when the patient attempts some

voluntary movement. Other features include scanning speech, dysmetria, past pointing, rebound phenomenon and diadokinesia. (Ganong 225)

46. **Ans. A:** An abstract thought is converted to a movement by integration in cortical association areas first. Then it is relayed to the basal ganglia, lateral cerebellum, premotor and motor cortex. (Ganong 205)

47. **Ans. B:** Initiation of muscular movements is a function of basal ganglia. Neurons here discharge even before movement begins. They are involved in planning and programming of movement. (Ganong 218)

48. **Ans. B:** Sensory inputs relay in the thalamic nuclei before projecting to widespread areas in the cortex to cause an alert, aroused response. Nuclei concerned with efferent control mechanism receive input from basal ganglia, cerebellum and project to the motor cortex. They are concerned with planning and execution of an idea. (Ganong 195, 205)

49. **Ans. B:** During the aware state, the cortical neurons are associated with a more rapid firing rate, the thalamic neurons are depolarized and fire tonically at rapid rates. (Ganong 200)

50. **Ans. C:** Thalamocortical oscillations form cortical dipoles and are responsible for resting EEG. (Ganong 200)

51. **Ans. B:** Anterior hypothalamus or preoptic area help raise the temperature set points by increasing thyroid activity, vasoconstriction. Posterior hypothalamus produce decrease in temperature set points by vasodilation, sweating. (Ganong 259)

52. **Ans. C:** Transection of brainstem at the superior border of the pons is called decerebration. The spasticity is due to increase in the gamma efferent nerves and increase in general excitability of motor neuron pool. Righting reflexes are integrated at the level of midbrain and will be consequently absent in a decerebrate preparation. (Ganong 216)

53. **Ans. D:** Right inferior temporal in right handed individuals help in storage and recognition of faces. Lesions in this area cause prosopagnosia, the inability to recognize faces. Medial temporal lobes are involved in encoding events for events or explicit memories. (Ganong 275)

54. **Ans. C:** Optical righting reflex, Placing and hopping reactions are integrated in the cerebral cortex. They help to maintain and support posture in response to various visual, exteroceptive and proprioceptive cues. Six directions : up is cortex, below dorsal column, sides ears and vestibular apparatus, back cerebellum and front eyes help maintain the posture and balance. (Ganong 211)

55. **Ans. E:** Golgi tendon organs are the receptor of the inverse stretch reflex. It helps to regulate velocity of muscle contraction, muscle length and muscle force. Muscle spindle is the receptor of muscle stretch and length. The pathways are dorsal and ventral spinocerebellar carry these signals from the body, cuneocerebellar from the head and neck. New learning proprioceptive signals like playing a casio are carried by the olivocerebellar tracts. (Ganong 131-133, 225)

56. **Ans. D:** Hemiballismus are involuntary movements that are failing, intense and violent. Caudate nucleus lesions produce rapid, involuntary "dancing" movements called chorea.

57. **Ans. B:** Parkinson's disease has a triad of akinesia, bradykinesia (rigidity and

tremors), hyperkinetic features. (Ganong 219)

58. **Ans. B:** Adminstration of L-dopa (levo-dopa) crosses the blood brain barrier and helps repair the dopamine deficiency. (Ganong 220)

59. **Ans. C:** The direction of Nystagmus is given by the direction of the fast component of the oscillation. The characteristic jerky movement of the eye observed at the start and end of a period of rotation is called nystagmus. The direction of nystagmus is opposite to the direction of nystagmus to maintain visual fixation (Vestibular ocular reflex). (Ganong 186)

60. **Ans. A:** Transection of brainstem at the superior border of the pons is called decerebration. The spasticity is due to increase in the gamma efferent nerves and increase in general excitability of motor neuron pool. Righting reflexes are integrated at the level of midbrain and will be consequently absent in a decerebrate preparation. Visual righting reflex are integrated in cerebral cortex and will be absent in a thalamic animal. Decortication is removal of cerebral cortex and produces little motor deficit in many mammals. Rigidity occurs due to loss of cortical areas inhibits γ efferent discharge in reticular formation. Hopping and placing reaction are absent in a decorticate preparation. (Ganong 216)

61. **Ans. D:** Reticular formation in the medulla and midbrain is concerned with regulation of heart rate, blood pressure and respiration. Descending pathways are involved in supraspinal control of stretch reflexes and posture control. The ascending RAS is concerned with consciousness and sleep. (Ganong 195,196)

62. **Ans. C:** The respiration becomes slower and tidal volume greater when the vagi are intact. Prolonged inspiratory spasms that resemble breath-holding is called Apneusis, when vagi are cut and Pneumotaxic centre is destroyed. They play a role in switching between inspiration and expiration. (Ganong 676)

63. **Ans. B:** Bitemporal hemianopia (half blindness). Lesions affecting the optic chiasm, such as pituitary tumors expanding the sella turcica, cause destruction of the fibers from both nasal hemiretinas and produce heteronymous (opposite side of the visual fields) hemianopia. (Ganong 170)

64. **Ans. C:** A δ fibers conduct pain, cold, touch. C fibers conduct pain, temperature, mechanoreception, reflex responses. (Ganong 61)

65. **Ans. D:** The fiber thickest is A α with diameter of 12-20 mm and conduction velocity of 70-120 m/sec. They convey proprioception, somatic motor impulses. (Ganong 61)

66. **Ans. C:** True visceral pain is carried by C fibers to the spinal cord (Ganong 144). It is poorly localized, nauseating and frequently associated with sweating and changes in blood pressure. (Ganong 144)

67. **Ans. D:** Acetylcholine is distributed throughout the CNS. There is a large projection from the nucleus of the basalis of Meynert and adjacent nuclei to the amygdale and the entire neocortex. These projections are involved in motivation, perception and cognition. They are lost in Alzeimer's disease. (Ganong 269)

68. **Ans. D:** Alpha rhythm is seen in awake with eyes closed, showing a relaxed but aware state. Beta rhythm or desynchronized

rhythm is seen when awake with eyes open showing an alert and aroused state. (AK Jain 1012)

69. **Ans. B:** Broca's area of speech is the motor speech area and Wernicke's area of speech is the sensory area. Broca's aphasia produces telegraphic speech, Wernicke's aphasia is a form of fluent aphasia, where the patient speaks many words without understanding, new words (Neologisms). (Ganong 278, 279)

70. **Ans. C:** Frequency of alpha wave is 8-12 Hz, beta waves is 14-30 Hz, Theta 4-7 z, Delta 1-4 Hz. (AK Jain 1012)

71. **Ans. D:** Marked variation in local blood flow occurs with changes in brain activity. In subjects who are awake but at rest, blood flow is greatest in the premotor and frontal regions as this part of brain is believed to be concerned with decoding and analyzing afferent input with intellectual activity. (Ganong 621)

72. **Ans. C:** First order neurons is from periphery to post horn cells. Second horn cells from post horn cells to the thalamus and third order neurons from thalamus to cortex. (Ganong 140)

73. **Ans. A:** Wallerian degeneration is the retrograde destruction occurring in nerve fibers after injury. (AK Jain 141, 153)

74. **Ans. B:** The oscillation is the intention tremor of cerebellar disease. It is absent at rest (unlike the temor of Parkinsonism). It appears whenever the patient attempts to perform some voluntary action. (Ganong 224)

75. **Ans. C:** Basal ganglia are also involved in processes in which an abstract thought is converted to voluntary action. (Ganong 218)

76. **Ans. D:** Somatosensory area (S1) is represented in the postcentral gyrus. There is detailed localization of fibers from various parts of the body, in form of columns similar to the occipital cortex. (Ganong 141)

77. **Ans. A:** Touch, pain and temperature pathways are the sensations carried by anterolateral spinothalamic tracts that project to mesencephalic reticular formation and nonspecific thalamic nuclei that project to the somatosensory cortex, Brodmann's area 1, 2 and 3. (Ganong 140, 141)

78. **Ans. A:** Unconscious kinesthetic sensation are carried from anterior spinal horns by ventral and dorsal spinocerebellar tracts. (Ganong 225)

79. **Ans. C:** Conduction velocity in nerve fibers of Aα is 70-120 m/s as they conduct information of proprioception that needs to be relayed quickly to the brain. (Ganong 61)

80. **Ans. D:** Median eminence is funnel shaped and serves as an area where all releasing factors and hormones find a way to enter pituitary from the hypothalamus. (Ganong 400)

81. **Ans. C:** The cortical representation of each body part is proportionate in size to the skill with which part is proportionate in size to the skill, fine voluntary movements. Areas involved in speech and hand movements are large in the cortex. (Ganong 207)

82. **Ans. A:** Parkinsonism is characterized by a triad of rigidity, tremor (hyperkinesias) and mask like facies (hypokinesia). Rigidity is of leadpipe or cogwheel type. (Ganong 219)

83. **Ans. B:** Motor areas give rise to pyramidal tracts, whose stimulation produces prompt discrete movement. It is present in the precentral gyrus. (Ganong 207)

84. **Ans. A:** The ventricles do not receive blood supply from the parasympathetic

vagi and are supplied by the sympathetic nerves from stellate ganglion. The SAN develops from the structures on right side of embryo and AVN from structures on the left. (Ganong 550)

85. **Ans. A:** Cerebral blood flow is regulated at arterial pressure of 65-140 mm Hg. Noradrenergic discharge helps to regulate pressure between 65-200 mm Hg (plateau phase is extended to right). Vasodilator hydralazine and ACE inhibitor captopril reduce the length of the plateau. (Ganong 610)

86. **Ans. D:** Fast pain is conveyed by Aδ and slow visceral pain by C fibers. (Ganong 61)

87. **Ans. C:** Type I afferent is from Nuclear bag fiber. Type II innervate nuclear chain fiber and have flower spray ending. They control the slow dynamic and static response of stretch reflex respectively. (Ganong 13)

88. **Ans. C:** Extraocular, hand muscles are white muscles, specialized for fine, skilled movements. Antigravity, back muscles are red muscles adapted for long, slow posture maintaining contraction. (Ganong 73)

89. **Ans. B:** Dopamine causes schizophrenia like symptoms, its concentration are required for planning and programming in basal ganglia. Serotonin neurons discharge rapidly in wakeful state and are involved in migraine, improved moods and circadian rhythms. Noradrenaline elevate mood and vigilance, secretion of vasopressin and oxytocin. (Ganong 267)

90. **Ans. B:** Stretch reflex is a monosynaptic reflex with a synaptic delay of 0.5 ms. (Ganong 131)

91. **Ans. A:** Due to cortical plasticity, limb cortical area responds to touching of face in cases of war amputees (Phantom limb pain). This shows that despite the law of projection sensory units to cortex have extensive convergence and divergence. (Ganong 142)

92. **Ans. D:** Continuous type of capillary is found in muscle, brain. Fenestrated capillaries are found in endocrine glands, intestinal villi and part of kidney for exchange of hormones, nutrients and excretory products. (Ganong 581)

93. **Ans. C:** Weber-Fechner law states that magnitude of sensation felt is proportionate to the log of intensity of stimulus. (Ganong 127)

94. **Ans. D:** Stretch reflexes, supporting reaction are integrated in spinal cord. Labyrinthine and Tonic neck reflex are integrated in the medulla. Optical righting reflexes, placing and hopping reactions are integrated in cerebral cortex. (Ganong 211)

95. **Ans. B:** Medial or ventral pathways and neurons are concerned with the control of muscles of the trunk and proximal portions of the limbs, whereas lateral pathways are concerned with the control of the muscles in the distal portion of the limbs. Axial muscles are concerned with posture, equilibrium and tone, distal limb muscles are involved in fine, skilled movements. (Ganong 200)

96. **Ans. B:** Acetylcholine is the neurotransmitter of vagus nerves that mediates the cephalic reflex (Choice C, i.e., gastric secretion in response to sight and smell of food and responses of gastric secretion to emotions and glucose (after food). Emotion of happiness increases gastric secretion but emotion of grief and depression decrease it. Other neurotransmitters involved are histamine, PGE_2. (Ganong 497)

97. **Ans. B:** All or none law states that when a sub threshold stimulus produce no change

in action potential. An action potential results once threshold intensity of stimuli is reached. Further increases in stimuli does not result increase in magnitude in action potential. (Ganong 52)

98. **Ans. A:** Lateral hypothalamic area (LHA) is the hunger centre. Ventral medial (VM) nucleus is the satiety centre. Stimulation of VM nucleus or LHA produces satiety. (Ganong 240)

99. **Ans. D:** Noradrenergic impulses produces thick viscous salivary secretion (α_1) and amylase rich secretion (β); contraction of radial iris muscle-mydriasis (α_1) and relaxation of ciliary muscle (β_2), and glycogenolysis (α_1, β_2). (Ganong 229, 231)

100. **Ans. B:** Fast anterograde transport occurs at 400 mm/d along microtbules, slow anterograde transport at 0.5-10 mm/d. Retrograde transport in opposite direction occurs at 200 mm/d. (Ganong 53)

101. **Ans. C:** Renshaw cell are located in ventral horns of the spinal cord in association of motor neurons. Stimulation of Renshaw cell inhibits neighboring motor neurons in that it helps to focus or sharpen the signal, suppressing spread to adjacent neurons. (AK Jain 882)

102. **Ans. C:** Sleep spindles have frequency of 10-14 Hz in Stage 2 sleep. These are alpha like waves. (Ganong 198)

103. **Ans. B:** During the isometric relaxation phase the valves are closed, pressure continues to drop rapidly. Isovolumetric relaxation phase ends when the ventricular pressure falls below the atrial pressure and the AV valves open. (Ganong 568, 569)

104. **Ans. C:** Golgi tendon organ are receptors for inverse stretch reflex. Unlike the muscle spindles they are in series with the muscle fibers and are stimulated by both passive stretch and active contraction of muscle. It works as a transducer feedback mechanism to prevent excessive muscle regulating velocity of muscle contraction, length and force. (Ganong 135)

105. **Ans. A:** Golgi tendon organ are receptors for inverse stretch reflex. Unlike the muscle spindles, they are in series with the muscle fibers, and are stimulated by both passive stretch and active contraction of muscle. It works as a transducer feedback mechanism to prevent excessive muscle regulating velocity of muscle contraction, length and force. (Ganong 135)

106. **Ans. C:** Cerebral blood flow is regulated at arterial pressure of 65-140 mm Hg. Noradrenergic discharge helps to regulate pressure between 65 and 200 mm Hg (plateau phase is extended to right). Vasodilator hydralazine and ACE inhibitor captopril reduce the length of the plateau. (Ganong 610)

107. **Ans. D:** Transection of brainstem at the superior border of the pons is called decerebration. The spasticity is due to increase in the gamma efferent nerves and increase in general excitability of motor neuron pool. Righting reflexes are integrated at the level of midbrain and will be consequently absent in a decerebrate preparation. (Ganong 216)

108. **Ans. D:** Blood sugar is maintained at a steady level almost to the end. It is formed from liver from amino acid residues, glycerol from fats and lactic acid from partial catabolism of muscle glycogen. (AK Jain 646)

109. **Ans. B:** Impulses pass normally in one direction only, i.e., from synaptic junction or receptor along the axon to their termination called *Orthodromic conduction.*(AK Jain 148, 341) Axon reflex is a response in which impulses

are initiated in sensory nerves by injury and are relayed antidromically down other branches of sensory nerves. Red reaction, wheal (swelling), flare (redness spreading from site of reaction) are the three components of triple response. (Ganong 629)

110. **Ans. D:** Spike duration is maximum in C fibers about 2 msec. The spike duration is least in A fibers about 0.4-1 msec. (AK Jain 138)

111. **Ans. A:** A α fibers have a diameter of 12-20 mm and carry fastest impulses of proprioception @ 70-120 mm/sec. (Ganong 61)

112. **Ans. B:** Superior colliculi is the integrating midbrain centre for light reflex. (Ganong 157)

113. **Ans. C:** Pendular knee jerk is seen in cerebellar disease. (Ganong 225)

114. **Ans. B:** Gag reflex or Uvular reflex has afferent IX and efferent X nerve. (AK Jain 873)

115. **Ans. C:** Sleep spindles have frequency of 10-14 Hz in Stage 2 sleep. These are alpha like waves. (Ganong 198)

116. **Ans. A:** Even the brainstem can withstand hypoxia for ten minutes whereas other parts of the brain can resist it for only ten seconds. (AK Jain 149, 150)

117. **Ans. B:** Gag reflex or uvular reflex: Afferent is the IX nerve and efferent is X nerve. (AK Jain 873)

118. **Ans. C:** Nigrostriatal neurons are rich in dopamine. They are inhibitory in nature. Acetylcholine discharge is excitatory. Balance between the two is lost in Parkinsonism. (Ganong 220)

119. **Ans. A:** Serotonin and Glutamate are excitatory neurotransmitters. Glutamate forms 7% of excitatory neurotransmitter. Serotonin has a role for mood elevation. Glutamate is involved in NMDA receptors and long-term potentiation. (Ganong 110)

120. **Ans. A:** GABA receptor are of 3 types. They increase in Cl^- influx and K^+ efflux to hyperpolarize all neurons. They are potentiated by Benzodiazepines, e.g., diazepam and is used as sedatives and muscle relaxants. (Ganong 112)

121. **Ans. A:** Rheobase is the minimum voltage required to produce an action potential. Chronaxie is the time double of the rheobase required to stimulate. A less excitable tissue will more time and voltage to be stimulated. (AK Jain 38)

122. **Ans. A:** Cortex of long vertical columns is present in the optical cortex and in the somatosensory cortex. *Complex cells* respond to a linear stimuli of light that is moved laterally. Simple cells of the cortex are responsive to linear stimuli like bars of light, lines or edges that have only a particular position. Wheras bipolar cells are cells of the inner nuclear layer of retina (layer 6). (AK Jain 1154)

123. **Ans. A:** Decrease in excitability is manifested by stimulation of parasympathetic system (Negative bathmotropic). (AK Jain 338)

124. **Ans. A:** Both fibrous and protoplasmic astrocytes send processes to blood vessels where they induce capillaries to form tight junctions that form blood brain barrier. (AK Jain 394-395)

125. **Ans. C:** Slow muscle units are innervated by small slowly conducting motor units and fast units by large, rapidly conducting motor neuron (Size principle). (Ganong 76)

126. **Ans. B:** Purkinje fibers have a conduction rate of 4 m/s. Atrial pathways @ 1 m/s and SAN 0.05 m/s. (Ganong 551)

127. **Ans. B:** Rhomberg's sign is positive when tracts of proprioception conscious and unconscious are lesioned. They include dorsal and spinocerebellar tracts respectively. (AK Jain 922)

128. **Ans. C:** The Golgi tendon reflex is also called as Inverse stretch reflex. It also is a protective reflex and regulates muscle tension. It is integrated in the spinal cord and involves irradiation of the stimuli to recruit a number of motor neurons. On stronger stimuli occurs extension of the opposite limb called crossed extensor reflex. However, the stretch reflex is best known monosynaptic reflex in the body. It is a "fundamental" reflex which plays a role in control of body postures. (AK Jain 905, 907, 898)

129. **Ans. C:** CSF constituents are Na 147 K 2.9 Cl 113 Glucose 64. Plasma constituents are Na 150 K 4.6 Cl 99 Glucose 100 (meq/kg H_2O). Cl- concentration is higher in plasma. (Ganong 615)

130. **Ans. C:** Water, CO_2 and O_2 penetrate the brain with ease. CO_2 is twenty times more diffusible than O_2. So do the lipid soluble free forms of steroid hormones, protein bound forms do not. (Ganong 617, 618)

131. **Ans. C:** Broca's area is the motor speech area. Lesions produce telegraphic speech.

132. **Ans. D:** Water, CO_2 and O_2 penetrate the brain with ease. CO_2 is twenty times more diffusible than O_2. So do the lipid soluble free forms of steroid hormones, protein bound forms do not. The easy penetration of CO_2 contrasts with the slow penetration of H^+ and HCO_3^- and has physiological significance in respiration. (Ganong 617, 618)

133. **Ans. B:** The width of A bands is constant, whereas the Z lines move closer together when the muscle contracts and farther apart when it is stretched. (Ganong 69)

134. **Ans. B:** Athetoid movements are slow writhing movements. They are involuntary in nature and a manifestation of hyperkinesis. (Ganong 218)

135. **Ans. D:** The general properties of reflexes are adequate stimulus to produce a response, alpha motor neuron being the final common pathway, habituation, sensitization, fatiguability. (AK Jain 908)

136. **Ans. D:** *Unmyelinated* C fibers are of two types according to Erlanger and Gasser's classification. The dorsal root C fibers conduct pain, touch, temperature and impulses generated by cutaneous receptors. The sympathetic C fibers are *postganglionic sympathetic* nerve fibers. *Unmyelinated* C fibers conduct at the rate of 0.5 – 2 m/sec and 0.7–2.3 m/sec, respectively

137. **Ans. D:** Sherrington described hypothalamus as the head ganglion of the ANS. Stimulation produces autonomic responses. (Ganong 238)

138. **Ans. B:** Axon reflex is a response in which impulses are initiated in sensory nerves by injury and are relayed antidromically down other branches of sensory nerves. Red reaction, wheal (swelling), flare (redness spreading from site of reaction) are the three components of triple response. (Ganong 629)

139. **Ans. B:** When intracranial pressure is elevated to more than 33 mm Hg over a short period, cerebral blood flow is significantly reduced. The resultant ischemia stimulates the vasomotor area and systemic blood pressure rises. This is called Cushing reflex and helps to maintain the cerebral blood flow. (Ganong 621)

140. **Ans. C:** O_2 consumption of brain is 46 ml/min and 3.3 ml/100 g/min. (Ganong 615)

141. **Ans. C:** O_2 consumption of brain is 46 ml/ min and 3.3 ml/100 g/min. (Ganong 615)

142. **Ans. D:** Pneumotaxic centre is in the medial parabrachial and Kolliker-fuse nuclei in dorsolateral pons. It plays a role in switching between inspiration and expiration. When this centre is damaged the inspiration becomes prolonged and spasmodic that resembles breath-holding (apneusis–under control of apneustic centre). (Ganong 676)

143. **Ans. C:** Hypoxia stimulates the carotid and aortic bodies: the peripheral chemoreceptors especially in high altitude acclamatisation. CO_2 acts via CSF and brain interstitial fluid stimulation. (Ganong 677)

144. **Ans. C:** The muscle of arteries and arterioles is innervated by noradrenergic nerve fibers which are constrictor in function, and in some instances by cholinergic fibers which dilate the vessels. (Ganong 579)

145. **Ans. D:** Thalamocortical form oscillating dipoles that is the origin of EEG. (Ganong 200)

146. **Ans. C:** Signs of upper motor neuron paralysis is hypertonicity, positive Babinski's sign, i.e., on stimulating the outer edges of the sole of the foot with firm tactile stimulus produces first an upward movement, i.e., dorsiflexion of the great toe and fanning out abduction of small toes. This is due to a flexor withdrawal response. The causes are deep sleep, infants below one year of age, pyramidal tract lesions and Cheyne-Stokes respiration due to hypoxia. (Ganong 206)

147. **Ans. A:** Reticular activating system causes an alert, aroused, awake response. (Ganong 195)

148. **Ans. D:** Water, CO_2 and O_2 penetrate the brain with ease. CO_2 is twenty times more diffusible than O_2. So do the lipid soluble free forms of steroid hormones, protein bound forms do not. (Ganong 617,618)

149. **Ans. D:** Removal of the spinal cord and hind brain from influences of the rest of the brain by transaction of the brainstem at the superior border of the pons is called decerebration. (Ganong 213)

150. **Ans. A:** The retinohypothalamic pathway pass from the optic chiasm to the suprachiasmatic nuclei that regulate the sleep wake cycles, activity patterns, pineal hormone secretion, ACTH hormones. (Ganong 238)

151. **Ans. D:** Auditory pathways start from spiral ganglia that innervate hair cells of VIII nerve entering the medulla and ends in ventral and dorsal *cochlear nuclei*. These relay second order neurons to *superior olive and trapezoid body*. These pass up via lateral nucleus to *inferior colliculi*, projecting and relaying to *reticular formation, medial geniculate body in thalamus and primary auditory cortex* (Area 41) located in temporal cortex. (A K Jain 1104-05, 1128)

152. **Ans. D:** Corneal, Plantar and abdominal reflexes are superficial reflexes. Deep or tendon reflexes are knee and biceps reflex. Organic reflexes are deglutition (swallowing), defecation, suckling, grasping and micturition reflex. (AK Jain 906, 1068)

153. **Ans. D:** Area 6 is premotor area. Area 4 is primary motor area. Ischemia in Brodman's area 4 leads to monoplegia (paralysis of one limb). (AK Jain 940)

154. **Ans. D:** Postural reflexes integrated in the spinal cord are the spinal reflexes or stretch reflexes, e.g., Positive and Negative supporting reaction. (AK Jain 978, 983)

155. **Ans. A:** Conditioned reflex are an important type of learning. These require formation of new connections at the cortical and subcortical level. They cannot be built up in decorticate animal. (AK Jain 1070)

156. **Ans. D:** Rubrospinal, tectospinal, reticulospinal, vestibulospinal tracts are extrapyramidal tracts, they are facilitatory over flexor muscle tone, mediate reflex postural movements in response to visual and auditory stimuli. (AK Jain 941)

157. **Ans. D:** Alpha rhythm is seen in awake with eyes closed, showing a relaxed but aware state. Beta rhythm or desynchronized rhythm is seen when awake with eyes open showing an alert and aroused state. (AK Jain 1017)

158. **Ans. A:** The paleocerebellum evolved next and is represented by anterior lobe and parts of posterior lobe, e.g., pyramid and uvula. These represent spinocerebellum and receives proprioceptive input from lower part of body. The cerebellum is attached to the cerebral cortex like a three pin plug: superior, inferior and middle peduncles. (AK Jain 989)

159. **Ans. A:** Frequency of alpha wave is 8-12 Hz, beta waves is 14-30 Hz, Theta 4-7 z, Delta 1-4 Hz. Theta also occurs in early sleep, beta in infants, delta during overbreathing or organic brain diseases seen in awake state. (AK Jain 1012)

160. **Ans. A:** Homonymous upper quadrantanopia is also called "pie in the sky" are seen as some fibers relay to the temporal lobe from the lateral geniculate body. (AK Jain 1128)

161. **Ans. C:** End plate potential or graded potential is a nonpropagating in nature, confined to a local response. It can be either depolarizing or hyperpolarizing response. It has no refractory period or threshold and does not obey all or none response. (AK Jain 159)

162. **Ans. B:** Sensory area is located in the post central gyrus. The cortically processed sensations are stereognosis, two-point discrimination. Two-point discrimination (or the ability to distinguish between two adjacent stimuli on the skin) is a cortical sensation that is tested by a Weber's compass. The sole of the feet and back are least sensitive areas. Here the sensory units are large and widely spaced. (AK Jain 912, 921, 931)

163. **Ans. D:** Ionic basis of EPSP is explained on the following basis: The released excitatory transmitters bind to appropriate postsynaptic receptors and cause opening of "chemically" gated (Na+ or Ca++) ion channels in the subsynaptic membrane of the post synaptic cell. (AK Jain 879)

164. **Ans. D:** NREM sleep results probably due to stoppage of discharge of serotonin secreting neurons of midline *raphe nuclei* of pons and medulla. (*Raphe* means line of junction of the two halves of a structure which is formed in the embryo from bilateral rudiments. (AK Jain 1019)

165. **Ans. C:** Tremor of cerebellar disease appears when the patient attempts some voluntary movement. Other features include scanning speech, dysmetria, past pointing, rebound phenomenon and diadokinesia. (Ganong 225)

166. **Ans. D:** Micturition (control of urinary bladder) and defecation are autonomic reflexes that are lost in spinal shock. It is called Shock because none of the motor, sensory or autonomic systems of the body are functional. The deep tendon reflexes are exaggerated, i.e., of upper motor neuron type due to loss of inhibition from the higher centres. (AK Jain 959)

167. **Ans. D:** C fibers are of two types according to Erlanger and Gasser's classification. The dorsal root C fibers conduct pain, touch, temperature and impulses generated by cutaneous receptors. The sympatheric C fibers are postganglionic sympathetic nerve fibers. Unmyelinated C fibers conduct at the rate of 0.5 – 2 m/sec and 0.7–2.3 m/sec, respectively. (AK Jain 149)

168. **Ans. D:** Increase in concentration of ECF by 2000 times from 10^{-7}moles/l to 2×10^{-4} moles/l. Calcium binds to troponin C causing tropomyosin to move laterally exposing the binding sites for myosin on actin. Hence muscular contraction occurs. (AK Jain 168)

169. **Ans. A:** GABA receptor are of 3 types. They increase in Cl^- influx and K^+ efflux to hyperpolarize all neurons. They are potentiated by Benzodiazepines, e.g., diazepam and is used as sedatives and muscle relaxants (Ganong 112). Inhibitory amino acids, e.g., GABA *(Gamma-aminobutyric acid*) are inhibitory in cerebellum and spinal cord. (AK Jain 1076, 1081)

170. **Ans. C:** Exterioreceptors are concerned with the perception of external environment, e.g., pressure, touch, pain, temperature. These are Pacinian corpuscle, Merkel's disc, Ruffini's end organ, naked nerve endings. (AK Jain 889)

171. **Ans. D:** Negative Babinski's sign, i.e., on stimulating the outer edges of the sole of the foot with firm tactile stimulus produces first and downward movement, i.e., plantar flexion of the great toe and adduction of small toes. This is due to a grasping response. This is to enable normal walking. The causes are deep sleep, infants below one year of age, pyramidal tract lesions and Cheyne-Stokes respiration due to hypoxia. (Ganong 206)

172. **Ans. C:** Reverberatory circuits are branched pathways which turn back on themselves allowing activity to strike back. They are seen in brain and spinal cord, and causes prolonged bombardment of motor neurons prom a single stimulus and result in prolonged response. This is called *Long-term potentiation* for formations of memory neural proteins. (AK Jain 906)

173. **Ans. A:** The axons of presynaptic neurons divide into many branches to end on many post synaptic neuron, e.g., motor neuron of muscle. (AK Jain 883)

174. **Ans. D:** Parkinson's disease is caused by decrease in dopamine in the nigrostriatal system. Athetosis is slow writhing snake like movements seen in lesion of lentiform nucleus. Chorea is fast, dancing like movement due to lesions of caudate nucleus of the basal ganglia. Hemiballismus are violent movements of half side of the body due to lesions in subthalamic nuclei. All are involuntary in nature. They may be controlled by Dopamine agonists. (AK Jain 1028, 1030)

175. **Ans. B:** Reinforcement and repetition activate the reverberatory Papez circuits to form neural proteins (*synthesized by RNA*) in development of long-term memory (LTP: Long-term potentiation). (AK Jain 1071, 2)

176. **Ans. B:** The flocculonodular lobe is functionally related to the vestibular apparatus and therefore called the vestibulocerebellum. It is concerned with control of body posture and equilibrium (AK Jain 990). Lesions of flocculonodular lobe leads to incordination or ataxia. Other features of cerebellar disease include Tremor that appears when the patient attempts some voluntary movement. Other features include scanning speech, dysmetria, past pointing, rebound phenomenon and diadokinesia. (Ganong 225)

177. **Ans. D:** Animals with diencephalic lesion, i.e., transaction of the brainstem immediately above the thalamus cause remarkable reaction of *sham rage,* i.e., only intense somatic (motor) and autonomic changes (similar to those that occur in rage in a normal animal in response to mild stimuli) without emotion. (AK Jain 1059)

178. **Ans. C:** The vagus nerve innervates muscles of heart, pharynx, larynx and GIT and glands of thorax and abdomen. The afferent component of the nerve also brings information from receptor in thorax and abdomen. Stimulation of vagus constricts the pupil, decreases heart rate, contractility, dilates arterioles, constricts bronchial muscles, stimulates salivary gland secretion, contracts gallbladder, contracts detrusor muscle to cause micturition. (AK Jain 873, 955)

179. **Ans. A:** The osmoreceptors which initiate drinking in response to increased plasma osmolality are located in the *lateral preoptic area* of the anterior hypothalamus. (AK Jain 1039)

180. **Ans. D:** Respiratory alkalosis due to hyperventilation is characterized by an elevated arterial pH, a low CO_2 tension (hypocapnia), and a variable decrease in bicarbonate. (AK Jain 574)

181. **Ans. C:** CSF is on average 130 mm H_2O (10 mm Hg) in lateral lying position (range 100-200 mm H_2O). In sitting position CSF pressure is 200 mm H_2O higher than in the lying position. (AK Jain 392)

182. **Ans. C:** Inhibitory amino acids, e.g., GABA (*Gamma-aminobutyric acid*), glycine are inhibitory in cerebellum and spinal cord. (AK Jain 1076)

183. **Ans. B:** In posterior part of temporal cortex is the area that processes information that can convert into auditory forms of word. This sensory speech area. (AK Jain 1066)

184. **Ans. D:** Hippocampus helps in forming new memories. Damage to this area results in the loss of recall of recent events (explicit memories). (AK Jain 1072)

185. **Ans. B:** Primary auditory cortex (Area 41) lies in the superior portion of the temporal lobe located in the floor of the lateral cerebral sulcus. Here nerve impulses are perceived as sound, i.e., loudness, pitch, source and direction of sound are analysed here. (AK Jain 1105)

186. **Ans. D:** The motor cortex is divided into two zones: "Area 4γ" and "Area 4α". Area 4γ lie posteriorly, called Giganopyramidalis due to the presence of giant cells of Betz in layer V of this region. (AK Jain 934)

187. **Ans. C:** The basic structural and functional unit of the nervous system is the neuron. Billions and trillions of such neurons constitute the nervous system. (AK Jain 869)

188. **Ans. B:** Baroreceptors are stretch receptors in the walls of heart and blood vessels. They are stimulated by distension when the blood pressure in these structures rises. Their afferent fibers pass via glossopharyngeal and vagus nerves to the medulla. Most of them end at NTS (nucleus tractus solitarius). NTS whose excitation decreases the arterial blood pressure primarily and subsequently vasodilation, bradycardia and venodilation. (Ganong 607, 608)

189. **Ans. D:** NTS whose excitation decreases the arterial blood pressure primarily and subsequently *bradycardia,* vasodilation, and venodilation. (Ganong 607, 608)

190. **Ans. D:** Acetylcholine binds to nicotine receptors. D-tubocurare and snake venom Bungarotoxin causes muscular paralysis by inhibiting the events by neuromuscular transmission. (AK Jain 953,1077)

191. **Ans. A:** Lateral hypothalamic area (LHA) is the hunger centre. Ventral medial (VM) nucleus is the satiety centre. Destruction of VM nucleus or LHA produces hyperphagia. (Ganong 240)

192. **Ans. D:** The axis of the mitral and tufted cells pass posteriorly through the lateral intermediate olfactory striae to the olfactory cortex. Sniffing activates the piriform cortex and smells without sniffing activates the orbital frontal gyrus of frontal lobe. (Ganong 189)

193. **Ans. B:** The sound frequencies audible to humans range from about 20 to a maximum of 20,000 cycles per second (cps, Hz). Pitch discrimination is best in the 1000 to 3000 Hz range and is poor at high and low pitches. (Ganong 179)

194. **Ans. A:** Nociceptive stimuli are painful stimuli transmitted by free nerve endings. Pacinian corpuscles respond to pressure. Merkel's disc and Ruffini end respond to temperature. (Ganong 125)

195. **Ans. B:** Cerebral blood flow in gray matter in resting humans is 69 ml/100 g/min compared to 100 g/min in white matter. Variation in blood flow occurs with changes in brain activity. Monro Kelly Doctrine states that the volume of blood in the cranium must remain constant at any times. (AK Jain 384-389)

196. **Ans. D:** Oligodendrocytes are involved in myelin formation in CNS. Microglia are scavenger cells resembling tissue macrophages. Astrocytes are of two types. Fibrous are seen in white matter, protoplasmic with granular cytoplasm are found in gray matter. They form the blood brain barrier. (Ganong 63)

197. **Ans. B:** Baroreceptors are stretch receptors in the walls of heart and blood vessels. They are stimulated by distension when the blood pressure in these structure rises. Their afferent fibers pass via glossopharyngeal and vagus nerves to the medulla. Most of them end at NTS (nucleus tractus solitarius). NTS whose excitation decreases the arterial blood pressure primarily and subsequently vasodilation, bradycardia and venodilation. (Ganong 607, 608)

198. **Ans. B:** Decreased ST segment shows an increased sympathetic activity or faster ventricular repolarisation. Its normal duration is 0.04 to 0.08 sec. Remaining are effects of vagus. (AK Jain 305)

199. **Ans. A:** Tabes dorsalis is seen in tertiary syphilis affecting posterior column, Rhomberg's sign is positive. The patient sways when the eyes are closed (sensory ataxia). Sensation carried by the dorsal column are somatic localization, vibration, touch (pneumonic PSVT). (Ganong 140)

200. **Ans. C:** Petit mal epilepsy is a form of epilepsy in children characterized by abrupt loss of conciousness without falling or incontinence, lasting for a few seconds. Here convulsive movements are absent or confined to slight twitching. EEG shows 3 per second doublets, each consisting of a typical spike and rounded waves. (AK Jain 1015)

201. **Ans. C:** Eccrine glands are seen on palms and soles and are supplied by cholinergic fibers present in sympathetic nerves. Atropine inhibits secretion. They are responsible for thermal sweating due to rise in temperature, emotional states, exercise, vomiting and ingestion of spicy food (AK Jain 596)

202. **Ans. C:** Axon reflex is a response in which impulses are initiated in sensory nerves by injury and are relayed antidromically down other branches of sensory nerves. Red reaction, wheal (swelling), flare (redness spreading from site of reaction) are the

three components of triple response. (Ganong 629)

203. **Ans. A:** Planum temporal a portion of posterior temporal gyrus is involved in language related processing. In musicians it is larger on the left side. Mobile phones should, thus be held on the left side. (Ganong 184)

204. **Ans. C:** 15-20% of the fibers are uncrossed and are called anterior corticospinal. (AK Jain 940)

205. **Ans. C:** The regular alpha rhythm breaks to a desynchronized low voltage, of irregular waves associated with a sensory disturbance or alert awake response. Seen when eyes that are closed (alpha) are opened (beta). (AK Jain 1012)

206. **Ans. C:** End plate potential or graded potential is a nonpropagating in nature, confined to a local response. It can be either depolarizing or hyperpolarizing response. It has no refractory period or threshold and does not obey all or none response. (AK Jain 159)

207. **Ans. B:** Blood brain barrier is absent in areas called circumventricular organs, e.g., Area postrema, posterior pituitary, osmoreceptor OVLT, subfornical organ (thirst) and pineal glands, median eminence of hypothalamus. (AK Jain 394-5)

208. **Ans. A:** The maintenance of posture and balance is accomplished by means of complex interaction of neural networks in spinal cord, brainstem, midbrain, and cortex and are called postural reflexes. Postural reflexes integrated in the spinal cord are the spinal reflexes or stretch reflexes, e.g., Positive and Negative supporting reaction (AK Jain 978, 983). The flexor withdrawal response is a protective response to potentially damaging nociceptive stimuli. It is integrated in the spinal cord and involves irradiation of the stimuli to recruit a number of motor neurons. On stronger stimuli occurs extension of the opposite limb called crossed extensor reflex. (AK Jain 907)

209. **Ans. D:** Unmyelinated nerves conduct slowly as its conduction is a continuous process. Conduction in myelinated fibers is 50-100 times faster because of leaping of impulses from one node to the other. (AK Jain 147)

210. **Ans. C:** Muscle fibers contain many myofibrils. Each myofibril is 1-2 micrometer in diameter. Myofibrils are made up of two sets of protein filaments, *thick and thin* filaments. Each thin filament contains 300-400 actin molecules and 40-60 tropomyosin molecules. (AK Jain 165)

211. **Ans. C:** The maintenance of posture and balance is accomplished by means of complex interaction of neural networks in spinal cord, brainstem, midbrain and cortex and are called postural reflexes. Postural reflexes integrated in the spinal cord are the spinal reflexes or stretch reflexes, e.g., Positive and Negative supporting reaction (AK Jain 978, 983). The flexor withdrawal response is a protective response to potentially damaging nociceptive stimuli. It is integrated in the spinal cord and involves irradiation of the stimuli to recruit a number of motor neurons. On stronger stimuli occurs extension of the opposite limb called crossed extensor reflex. The Golgi tendon reflex is also called as Inverse stretch reflex. It also is a protective reflex and regulates muscle tension. However, the stretch reflex is best known monosynaptic reflex in the body. It is a "fundamental" reflex which plays a role in control of body postures. (AK Jain 898, 905, 907)

212. **Ans. D:** Brown-Sequard syndrome or hemi section of spinal cord leads to loss of proprioception, somatic localization, vibration on the same side. These are carried by dorsal column that cross in the medulla. Pain, temperature carried by spinothalamic side of opposite side is lost as these tract cross at the same level of cord. Motor loss occurs at the same side of the spinal column. (AK Jain 962)

213. **Ans. D:** If there is extensive soft tissue and muscle crushing or catabolism called *Crush syndrome*, myoglobin leaks into circulation, it gets precipitated into renal tubules damaging them. (AK Jain 410)

214. **Ans. D:** True thirst (increase in water intake) is always associated with a *decrease of ECF volume*, or *an increase in plasma osmolality* (Increase in sodium from interstitial compartment). An injection of hypertonic saline into the lateral hypothalamic area induces drinking. (AK Jain 1039-1040)

215. **Ans. D:** Posterioinferior cerebellar artery supplies the posterior lobe of the cerebellum involved in functions of spinocerebellum and neocerebellum. These include proprioceptive impulses and pain, temperature, touch sensation. It is concerned with control of axial muscles and neocerebellum with fine, ambulatory movements. (AK Jain 990)

216. **Ans. C:** Micturition (control of urinary bladder) and defecation are autonomic reflexes that are lost in spinal shock. It is called Shock because none of the motor, sensory or autonomic systems of the body are functional. (AK Jain 959)

217. **Ans. A:** Alzheimer's disease is characterized by progressive loss of memory and *cognitive* functions. It leads to dementia, aphasia, agnosia (inability to recognize objects). The condition is caused by loss of cholinergic neurons in cerebral cortex and hippocampus. (AK Jain 1073)

218. **Ans. A:** During depolarization Na influx occurs, repolarisation occurs due to potassium efflux, after depolarization is the phase of slow potassium efflux. (AK Jain 36-37)

219. **Ans. C:** CSF pH is 7.33 as compared to plasma 7.40. (AK Jain 389-393)

220. **Ans. D:** Glucose concentration is 50-85 mg% as compared to 100 mg % of plasma. Ca++ concentration in CSF is only 2.3 mEq/L as compared to 4.7 in plasma. K+ is 2.9 in CSF as compared to 4.6 mEq/L in plasma. (AK Jain 389-393)

221. **Ans. B:** Protein concentration in CSF is 20-30 mg % and in plasma is 6000 mg%. The CSF contains some urea and uric acid and creatinine. However, it is free from cholesterol. (AK Jain 389-393)

222. **Ans. D:** Osmolality of both plasma and CSF is 289 mOsm/g/water. (AK Jain 389-393)

223. **Ans. D:** The weakest current strength which can excite a tissue, if allowed to flow through it for an adequate time is called *Rheobase*. The length of time for which a current twice "rheobase" intensity must be applied to produce a response is called chronaxie. Chronaxie values have been used as an index of excitability. (AK Jain 38). Cardiac muscle is the most excitable tissue in the choices, thus has minimum time to elicit a response.

224. **Ans. C:** The term chemical transmission is applied to substances called neuro-transmitters. Neurotransmitters influence ion channels by changing the membrane potential, the action occurs within milli-seconds, changes induced are fast and direct, they can activate both postsynaptic and presynaptic receptors. Acetylcholine

is most ideal as a neurotransmitter and also it acts as a local hormone. Substance P is a polypeptide neurotransmitter, Serotonin or 5-HT is a biogenic amine. (AK Jain 1075)

225. **Ans. C:** Golgi tendon organs are found in series with muscle fibers and there are 3-25 muscle fibers per tendon organ. (AK Jain 905)

226. **Ans. B:** Nernst equation of resting membrane potential RT/nF (LOG E) n-valency t-temperature E : Electrochemical gradient. (AK Jain 31, 32)

227. **Ans. B:** Dysmetria is difficulty in accuracy as in past pointing in cerebellar disease. The movement is poorly carried out in direction, range and force, therefore the movements *overshoot* their intended mark. It results in loss of neural circuit required to control the duration and strength of a movement. (AK Jain 1002)

228. **Ans. A:** Normally, cerebrospinal fluid occupies 10% of the intracranial volume. CSF represents transcellular fluid, i.e., fluid in the lumen of structures lined by epithelium. It also includes sweat, pleural, peritoneal, synovial, intraocular (aqueous and vitreous humors) and pericardial fluids, bile and luminal fluid of the gut, thyroid and cochlea. Trancellular fluid volume is relatively small, about 1L=15 ml/kg of body weight or 1.5% of body weight. (AK Jain 389)

229. **Ans. A:** Amino acid neurotransmitters are excitatory neurotransmitters, e.g., Excitatory amino acids, e.g., Glutamic acid, Aspartic acid and Inhibitory amino acids, e.g., GABA *(Gamma-aminobutyric acid)*, glycine are inhibitory in cerebellum and spinal cord. (AK Jain 1076)

230. **Ans. B:** Ischemia susceptible neurons are B fibers (Erlanger and Gasser's classification) which are "preganglionic" autonomic nerve fibers. The least sensitive to hypoxia is C fibers or dorsal root peripheral nerves that carry pain, touch, temperature and conduct impulses generated by cutaneous nerves. Even the brainstem can withstand hypoxia for ten minutes whereas other parts of the brain can resist it for only ten seconds. (AK Jain 149, 150)

231. **Ans. D:** The 12 nerve is hypoglossal and is purely motor in nature and innervate muscles of the tongue. Another purely motor nerve is spinal accessory nerve. 7,9, 10 are mixed nerves. (AK Jain 873)

232. **Ans. A:** Isometric means same measure or length. An isometric contraction occurs when the ends of the muscle do not move during contraction, i.e., muscle contracts, but length of the muscle remains the same. The tension or force that develops is considerable and can be measured by a force transducer. An example of isometric contraction is contraction of arm muscles trying to push a wall. (AK Jain)

233. **Ans. A:**The synapse between two efferent neurons lies outside the CNS in a cell cluster called autonomic ganglia. The nerve fibers passing between the CNS and the ganglia are called preganglionic and from the ganglionic cells to the periphery are postganglionic fibers. The neurotransmitter released between pre and post ganglionic fibers is *acetylcholine*, whereas it varies between postganglionic and effector depending on the effector. (AK Jain 947)

234. **Ans. C:** Cerebral blood flow is regulated at arterial pressure of 65-140 mm Hg. Noradrenergic discharge helps to regulate pressure between 65-200 mm Hg (plateau phase is extended to right). Vasodilator hydralazine and ACE inhibitor captopril reduce the length of the plateau. (Ganong 610)

235. **Ans. C:** Cerebral blood flow is 750 ml/min or 50-60 ml/min/100 gm. Critical flow level is approximately 18 ml/min/100 gm as flow less than this produces unconsciousness. (AK Jain 384,385)

236. **Ans. A:** Oligodendocytes are involved in myelin formation in CNS. Microglia are scavenger cells resembling tissue macrophages. Astrocytes are of two types. Fibrous are seen in white matter, protoplasmic with granular cytoplasm are found in gray matter. They form the blood brain barrier. (Ganong 63)

237. **Ans. C:** The flocculonodular lobe is functionally related to the vestibular apparatus and therefore called the vestibulocerebellum. It is concerned with control of body posture and equilibrium. (AK Jain 990)

238. **Ans. D:** Axon originates from a somewhat thickened area of the cell body called Axon Hillock. It is here where propagated action potentials are generated. (AK Jain 140)

239. **Ans. C:** Prefrontal lobe lesion results in flight of ideas, difficulty in planning, distractibility. The other features include euphoria, a sense of well being, indifference to the environment, loss of recent memory, loss of attention and restlessness, emotional instability. These are due to loss of connections between frontal lobe and thalamus and the other cortical association fibers. (AK Jain 1054)

240. **Ans. B:** The area in the upper pons, in the medial parabrachial nucleus, contain both I and E neurons, called pneumotaxic centre. These are active in both phases of inspiration and expiration and modify the rhythmic discharge of the medullary respiratory centre. A new concept of pace maker neurons called Pre Botzinger complex is present. The chloride channels are responsible for the rhythmicity of respiration, it is believed. (AK Jain 467, 468)

241. **Ans. C:** Striated muscle contains alternating bands of dark highly refractile Anisotropic A band and light band that is of lower refractile material called I band. (AK Jain 162)

242. **Ans. C:** Planum temporale a portion of posterior temporal gyrus is involved in language related processing. In musicians it is larger on the left side. Mobile phones should, thus be held on the left side. (Ganong 184)

243. **Ans. A:** Complete transaction of the spinal cord leads to flaccid paralysis. During the recovery stage after about two or three weeks, there occurs paralysis of the upper motor neuron type, characterized by hypertonia, brisk hyperactive reflexes and positive Babinski's sign. (AK Jain 959)

244. **Ans. A:** Nerve impulses can travel only orthodromically at synapse as acetylcholine vesicles are present only in the presynaptic terminal. (AK Jain 148)

245. **Ans. D:** The tracts in the dorsal (posterior column) include fasciculus gracilis and fasciculus cuneatus. The lateral white columns lie between the anterior and posterior roots. The tracts include *lateral spinothalamic tract, dorsal (posterior) spinocerebellar and ventral (anterior) spinocerebellar tract*. The tract in ventral (anterior) white column are ventral (anterior) spinothalamic tract. These are ascending tracts. The descending motor tracts are rubrospinal, tectospinal, reticulospinal, vestibulospinal tracts. The vestibulospinal is an uncrossed tract that descend throughout the spinal cord, originating in the lateral vestibular nuclei. It has facilitatory control on the reflex activity of spinal stretch reflex and helps control tone in antigravity muscles to maintain posture and equilibrium. (AK Jain 913)

246. **Ans. D:** Red muscle fibers are slow muscle fibers as they are innervated by small, slow conducting motor neuron. These muscles respond slowly and are adapted for long, slow posture maintaining contractions, e.g., long muscles of limb and muscles of the back. These have moderate glycogen stores and low ATPase activity. (AK Jain 174,175).

247. **Ans. A:** Pontocerebellar convey motor impulses from motor cortex via pontine nuclei to cerebellum via middle cerebellar peduncle. The cerebellum is attached to the cerebral cortex like a three pin plug: superior, inferior and middle peduncles. Olivocerebellar tract conveys information for learning new movements. (AK Jain 993)

248. **Ans. D:** Separate receptors exist for the somatic sensations (touch, pressure, pain and temperature). Combination of these sensations produce an entirely different experience of new sensations called synthetic senses. These are itch, vibration sense, two-point discrimination. (AK Jain 931)

249. **Ans. D:** Golgi tendon organ are found at the musculotendon junction in series with muscle fibers. Ib efferent from golgi tendon organ arises to synapse at inhibitory neurons in spinal cord. They help in regulating the inverse stretch reflex. 1a fiber is the afferent from muscle spindle. (AK Jain 905)

250. **Ans. A:** The motor homunculus shows representation of the body as upside down. Trunk, then arm, then thumb and face. The latter have maximum representation. (AK Jain 934)

251. **Ans. C:** CSF is produced by choroids plexus and ventricular walls and blood vessels. 550 ml per day is the production. Flow from III to IV is via cerebral aqueduct. (AK Jain 389-93)

252 **Ans. A:** Area 6 is premotor area. Area 4 is primary motor area. Ischemia in Brodman's area 4 leads to monoplegia (paralysis of one limb). (AK Jain 940)

253. **Ans. D:** Uterine contraction under the influence of oxytocin helps in expulsion of the baby from the uterus. Platelet plugging is another example of positive feedback homeostasis that prevents further bleeding. An example of positive feedback that may even lead to death occurs during haemorrhage. (AK Jain 3,522)

254. **Ans. D:** Intrafusal fibers are of two types: Nuclear bag fibers, Nuclear chain fibers. NBG contain many nuclei in a dilated central area, Nuclear chain fibers have a single chain of nuclei lying in a chain. Intrafusal muscle fibers contain 2-13 muscle fibers enclosed in a connective tissue capsule. (AK Jain 898)

255. **Ans. B:** Blood brain barrier breaks down in injury or infection. Tumors develop blood vessels that lack projections to astrocytes. (AK Jain 394-395)

256. **Ans. A:** Thalamus is a great sensory relay station and integrating centre before relaying it to the cerebral cortex. They relay somesthetic sensations coming from opposite of the body, i.e., pain, proprioception, temperature. They also form a relay of auditory and visual impulses, impulses from reticular formation. All other sensations (general or special) pass through the thalamus and projected to the neocortex, whereas the smell pathways have no relay in the thalamus and there is no neocortical projection area for olfaction. (AK Jain 1009)

257. **Ans. B:** Endolymph is formed by stria vascularis and has an electrolyte concentration similar to ICF. It is present in the scala media. (AK Jain 967, 1113)

258. **Ans. A:** Corticospinal tract arise from the motor cortex in the precentral gyrus. The lateral corticospinal tract controls lateral muscles or fine manibulatory movement and medial or anterior corticospinal tract control *p*osture *e*quilibrium and *t*one (memorise as PET). (AK Jain 936)

259. **Ans. B:** Myotonia is a condition characterized by difficulty and slowness in relaxing muscle after voluntary effort. This is due to abnormalities on genes 7,17 or 19 chromosomes, which result in abnormalities of Na+ or Cl- channels. (AK Jain 177)

260. **Ans. C:** Calcium is required for exocytosis of acetylcholine from presynaptic neuron to the synaptic cleft. Muscle weakness is caused by antibodies against one of the calcium channels in the nerve endings at neuromuscular junction. (AK Jain 160)

261. **Ans. A:** Blood brain barrier is absent in areas called circumventricular organs, e.g., Area postrema, posterior pituitary, osmoreceptor OVLT, subfornical organ (thirst) and pineal glands. (AK Jain 394-395)

262. **Ans. A:** Sarcotubular system are a highly specialized system of internal conduction of depolarization within muscle fiber. It is made of T tubule or transverse tubule and Longitudinal sarcoplasmic reticulum. (AK Jain 164)

263. **Ans. D:** Type IV afferent does not exist. Type I afferent is from Nuclear bag fiber. Type II innervate nuclear chain fiber and have flower spray ending. They control the slow dynamic and static response of stretch reflex respectively. Alpha motor neuron is the final common pathway to extrafusal fibre for stretch reflex. Gamma motor neuron is motor supply to intrafusal fiber. (Ganong 13)

264. **Ans. D:** Swallowing reflex is a brainstem reflex controlled via vagus nerve. (AK Jain 213, 214)

265. **Ans. B:** Via α1 receptors localized (adrenergic) sweating occurs. Generalised (cholinergic) sweating occurs to manifest parasympathetic effect of the sweat gland. (AK Jain 955)

266. **Ans. B:** Corticospinal tract arise from the motor cortex in the precentral gyrus. The lateral corticospinal tract controls lateral or *distal* muscles or fine manibulatory movement and medial or anterior corticospinal tract control posture equilibrium and *t*one (memorise as PET). (AK Jain 936)

267. **Ans. A:** Thalamus is a great sensory relay station and integrating centre before relaying it to the cerebral cortex. They relay somesthetic sensations coming from opposite of the body, i.e., pain, proprioception, temperature. They also form a relay of auditory and visual impulses, impulses from reticular formation. All other sensations (general or special) pass through the thalamus and projected to the neocortex, whereas the smell pathways have no relay in the thalamus and there is no neocortical projection area for olfaction. (AK Jain 1009, 1092)

268. **Ans. C:** Voluntary control of respiration is via corticospinal tract arising from cortex ending at spinal motor neurons, innervating respiratory group of neurons. Stimulation of respiratory centre by increased activity in the motor cortex causes increase in ventilation during exercise. Corticohypothalamic pathway ending on medullary group of neurons mediate and modify voluntary control of espiration through effecs of emotions such as anger, grief, sexual responses, depression. (AK Jain 467)

269. **Ans. C:** Sympathetic stimulation causes arteriolar constriction via alpha1 and dilation via beta 2, ciliary muscle relaxation for far vision vis beta 2, *decreased gut motility* via alpha1, alpha2 and beta2, increases salivary secretion causing thick secretions via alpha1. (AK Jain 954,955)

270. **Ans. D:** Parkinson's disease is caused by decrease in dopamine in the nigrostriatal system. The caudate nucleus and putamen are called Corpus striatum or Neostriatum these relay to Globus pallidus, i.e., paleostriatum which sends impulses to subthalamic nuclei, substantia nigra. Lesions here produce Pakinsonism. (AK Jain 1028)

271. **Ans. D:** The archicerebellum is the first part to develop during evolution and is represented by *flocculonodular lobe*. It is functionally linked to vestibulocerebellum. It is concerned with posture, equilibrium and tone. The paleocerebellum evolved next and is represented by anterior lobe and parts of posterior lobe, e.g., pyramis and uvula. These represent spinocerebellum and receives proprioceptive input from lower part of body. Neocerebellum is the newest and comprises remaining parts of posterior lobe, i.e., declive, tuber. They receive inputs from pons via pontocerebellum. (AK Jain 989)

272. **Ans. B:** Deep cerebellum nuclei input is negative. The granule cell is always excitatory in the cerebellar neural circuit. The basket cell, golgi and purkinje cell are inhibitory. (AK Jain 993)

273. **Ans. D:** The reticular formation is in the brainstem (pons and medulla). The function of RAS is regulation of cardiorespiratory function and vomiting as it harbours both centres. Hunger and thirst are controlled by the hypothalamus. (AK Jain 985)

274. **Ans. C:** Thumbs, Finger tips occupy maximum area in the somatosensory cortex. Lips are next. Two point discrimination (or the ability to distinguish between two adjacent stimuli on the skin) is a cortical sensation that is tested by a Weber's compass. The sole of the feet and back are least sensitive areas. Here the sensory units are large and widely spaced. (AK Jain 912, 921)

275. **Ans. C:** Tolerance to pain or inhibition to pain, i.e., Analgesia occurs due to increase in threshold. (AK Jain 927)

276. **Ans. A:** The afferent for segmental stretch reflex is 1a or Aα afferent fibers innervating nuclear bag and chain fibers of intrafusal origin. (AK Jain 899)

277. **Ans. A:** Motor axons give off some collateral branches as they traverse the spinal cord towards the ventral root, and these collaterals make excitatory synaptic connections with interneurons called *Renshaw cell*, situated in the ventromedial part of the ventral horn. These *Renshaw cell* in turn send axons which make synaptic connections with the motor neurons. This is an example of feed forward inhibition. (AK Jain 882)

278. **Ans. B:** A fibers are most sensitive to pressure. C fibers are least sensitive. (A K Jain 149)

279. **Ans. B:** The cortical representation for control of micturition is paracentral lobule. In the brainstem they are two areas: Facilitatory area is located in the pontine region and posterior hypothalamus. Inhibitory area is located in the midbrain. (AK Jain 587)

280. **Ans. A:** Smell pathways have no relay in the thalamus and there is no neocortical projection area for olfaction. The smell receptors are in direct contact with the

external environment. The smell receptors are distant receptors (*telereceptors)* as well as *chemoreceptors*. Their adaptation is early and rapid. (AK Jain 1092)

281. **Ans. A:** Duration of action potential in skeletal muscle is 2-4 msec. Nerve fiber duration is 0.4 to 2 msec. Action potential in cardiac muscle lasts 300 msec. (AK Jain 167)

282. **Ans. B:** Corticobulbar fibers end near the motor neurons that innervate muscles of eye, face, tongue and throat. These fibers are the main source of control for voluntary movement of the muscles of head and neck. They arise from the motor cortex and control movement of opposite side of the body. (AK Jain 936)

283. **Ans. A:** Axon originates from a somewhat thickened area of the cell body called Axon Hillock. It is here where propagated action potentials are generated. (AK Jain 140)

284. **Ans. C:** Increase in CSF pressure from its normal level initially leads to *Bulbar Asphyxia* which stimulates vasomotor centre producing extracerebral vasoconstriction and increases arterial mean BP. However, marked increases in CSF pressure produces direct depression of vasomotor centre and compensatory mechanism fails leading to respiratory depression and deterioration of consciousness. (AK Jain 389)

285. **Ans. A:** Blood brain barrier applies to the barrier between blood and the brain tissue. The endothelial cells are surrounded by a continuous belt of tight junctions that do not permit substances of more than molecular weight of 2000 to pass. On the other hand, endothelial cells are covered by foot processes of astrocytes that allow substances with a MW of 40,000. (AK Jain 394-95)

286. **Ans. A:** The autonomic nervous system shows some exceptions. In adrenal medulla, preganglionic fibers directly supply the adrenal medulla, where the postganglionic neurons have lost their axons and become specialized for secretion directly in the blood stream. It is an endocrine gland not under the control of automomic system but controlled by the sympathetic preganglionic fibers. Aldosterone is secreted from the adrenal gland. (AK Jain 948)

287. **Ans. A:** Trigeminal nerve innervates muscle of mastication (efferent) and afferent brings sensations from receptors in skin and skeletal muscles of face, nose and mouth from teeth sockets. (AK Jain 873)

288. **Ans. A:** Complete transaction of brainstem below medulla or above the spinal cord, stops all respiration (apnoea). Apneustic respiration or arrest of respiration in inspiration is seen on sectioning at the level of mid pons along with removal of vagi. Cheyne's stoke respiration is a form of periodic breathing seen during physiological hyperventilation, high altitude, brain damage and left ventricular failure. (AK Jain 467, 482)

289. **Ans. C:** Reflexes integrated in the mid brain are righting reflexes. These are a chain of reactions that maintain normal standing position and keep the head upright. Tonic labyrinthine righting reflex occurs due to alteration in the position of the head relative to the horizontal plane. Hopping, Placing reaction and Optical righting reflexes are integrated at the level of cerebral cortex. (AK Jain 976-978)

290. **Ans. D:** Auditory pathways start from spiral ganglia that innervate hair cells of VIII nerve entering the medulla and ends in ventral and dorsal *cochlear nuclei*. These relay second order neurons to *superior olive and trapezoid body*. These pass up via lateral nucleus to *inferior colliculi*, projecting and relaying to *reticular formation, medial geniculate body in thalamus and primary auditory cortex* (Area 41). Superior colliculi serves as a

centre for visual reflexes, e.g., light reflex. (AK Jain 1104-05, 1128)

291. **Ans. B:** Fever develops when the thermostat is reset to a new point above 37°C. *Interleukin-1* is an endogenous pyrogen that are produced by endotoxin from bacteria that stimulate monocytes, macrophages, Kupfer cells. These enter the brain to produce prostaglandins from preoptic area of hypothalamus producing fever. Aspirin inhibits this synthesis of prostaglandins, decreasing fever. (AK Jain 596-97)

292. **Ans. B:** The receptor of hearing is the organ of corti which is located on the basilar membrane extending from apex to the base of the Cochlea. The receptor is lined by a single row of *inner hair cells* and three or four rows of *outer hair cells*. Inner hair cells are primary sensory cells and are responsible for fine auditory discrimination. The outer hair cells are responsible for detecting the presence of sound. (AK Jain 1102-03)

293. **Ans. B:** The cells in visual cortex respond to lines and edges in their receptive fields. *Complex cells* respond to a linear stimuli of light that is moved laterally. Simple cells of the cortex are responsive to linear stimuli like bars of light, lines or edges that have only a particular position. Wheras bipolar cells are cells of the inner nuclear layer of retina (layer 6). (AK Jain 1154)

294. **Ans. B:** The climbing fibers arise from cells in the inferior olivary nucleus. They establish a one to one connection with the Purkinje cell dendrites and *excite* to discharge. These are responsible to play a role in learning important motor skills. (AK Jain 993, 994)

295. **Ans. B:** Broca's area is located in inferior frontal gyrus. It processes information received from Wernicke's area and projects to motor cortex which initiates movements of the lips, tongue and larynx to produce speech. Thus it is the motor speech area. Lesions heart produces nonfluent aphasias or motor aphasia where there is *compromised language output*. Speech is slow and words hard to come by and are limited to 2 or 3 words. They may also be Agraphia or inability to write and difficulty in articulation without mental confusion. (AK Jain 1066)

296. **Ans. D:** The regular alpha rhythm breaks to a desynchronized low voltage, of irregular waves associated with a sensory disturbance or alert awake response. Seen when eyes that are closed (alpha) are opened (beta). (AK Jain 1012)

The activity of many dendritic units is *synchronized* by formation of current sinks and sources of parallel neural processes between the thalamus and cortex. (AK Jain 1014)

297. **Ans. B:** The flow of saliva in response to ringing of the bell (*conditioned stimulus)* is referred to as conditioned reflex. The introduction of food (unconditioned stimulus) into the mouth sets up a reflex salivation in a dog called unconditioned stimulus. (AK Jain 1069)

298. **Ans. C:** The sympathetic preganglionic fibers leave the spinal cod with ventral roots of spinal cord between first thoracic and second lumbar segment called thoracolumbar divison. The nerve fibers leaving the CNS from the brain and sacral portion of spinal cord is via III, VII, IX and X cranial nerves and second and fourth spinal nerves. Hollow viscera like stomach have dual innervation from both sympathetic and parasympathetic division: Hypogastric plexus. This enables a very fine degree of control over the effector organ. (AK Jain 946, 951, 953)

299. **Ans. D:** Axon reflex is an example of antidromic conduction. Impulses pass normally in one direction only, i.e., from synaptic junction or receptor along the axon to their termination called *Orthodromic conduction*. (AK Jain 148, 341)

CHAPTER 2

Special Senses

What is Important in Special Senses?

Optics of Vision, Receptor Function, Sense of Hearing

1. When you look at a near object, the:

A. Depth of field decreases

B. Diopteric power of the lens decreases

C. Medial recti contract

D. Tension of the zonular fibers increases

2. Sound waves in the ear travel in:

A. Air medium B. Solid medium

C. Liquid medium D. All of the above

3. The process of swallowing involves all of the following except:

A. Closure of the glotii

B. Involuntary relaxation of the upper oesophageal sphincter

C. Involuntary movements of the tongue against the palate

D. Esophageal peristalsis

CONSIDER THE FOLLOWING RECEPTORS

1. Meissner's corpuscles
2. Merkel's disc
3. Pacinian corpuscles

4. Among these, rapidly adapting touch receptors would include:

A. 1, 2 and 3 B. 1 and 2

C. 1 and 3 D. 2 and 3

5. A traveling nerve impulse does not depolarize the area immediately behind it, because:

A. It is hypertrophied

B. It is refractory

C. It is not self-propagating

D. The conduction is always orthodromic

6. Eye gets totally adapted to darkness in ……… minutes.

A. 2 B. 5

C. 10 D. 20

7. Bitter taste is mediated by action of:

A. Guanyl cyclase

B. G protein

C. Tyrosine kinase

D. Epithelial Na^+ channels

8. Itching is caused by stimulation of:

A. A α fibers

B. B fibers
C. C fibers
D. Dorsal root ganglia

9. **Which of the following taste buds help protect against the ingestion of certain plant poisons?**
A. Sweet taste buds
B. Bitter taste buds
C. Sour taste buds
D. Salt taste buds

10. **Why is sudden loud sound is more likely to damage the cochlea than a prolonged loud sound?**
A. The basilar fibers are sensitive to sudden sounds but adapt to prolonged sounds
B. A sudden sound carries more energy
C. The tympanic membrane becomes flaccid during prolonged loud sounds
D. The fluid pressure in the scala tympani can decrease greatly during prolonged sound

11. **A light having a monochromate colour stimulates the red cones about twice as much as the green cones. What is the colour of this monochromate light?**
A. Green B. Orange
C. Red D. Yellow
E. Blue

12. **Ruffini end organ is associated with sensation of:**
A. Pressure B. Cold
C. Heat D. Touch
E. None of the above

13. **Stapes rests in:**
A. Round window
B. Oval window
C. Tympanic membrane
D. Basilar membrane

14. **The cones in the eye are:**
A. Not responsible for colour vision
B. More sensitive to light than the rods
C. Associated with higher visual acuity than the rods
D. Dependent on Vitamin A for their function

15. **Visual acuity is:**
A. A measure of sensitivity of retina to light
B. Better using one eye that using both eyes
C. Better with central than with peripheral vision
D. Reduced in colour blind persons

16. **Which of the following statement is most correct?**
A. Taste buds are sensitive to all of the gustatory modalities
B. There are over ten well defined distinct gustatory modalities
C. Taste projection is at the foot of the postcentral gyrus
D. None of the above

17. **The attenuation reflex is due to:**
A. Contraction of tensor tympani
B. Contraction of stapedius
C. Contraction of tensor tympani and stapedius
D. Inward movement of oval window

18. **Crude touch sensations are carried by:**
A. Ventral spinothalamic tract
B. Lateral spinothalamic tract
C. Posterior column
D. Pyramidal tract

19. Most of the refraction that occurs in the eye occurs at the:

A. Anterior surface of cornea
B. Posterior surface of cornea
C. Anterior surface of lens
D. Posterior surface of lens

20. Which one of the following procedures is most likely to increase intraocular pressure of glaucoma patients?

A. Use of atropine
B. Decreased pressure in jugular vein
C. High dose of Vitamin C
D. Dark environment
E. Carbonic anhydrase inhibitors

21. Taste fibers relay in:

A. Geniculate ganglion
B. Gasserian ganglion
C. Petrous ganglion
D. Otic ganglion

22. An aged violin player can get a correct pitch only by touching his teeth to the vibrating instrument. He is most likely to damage:

A. Inner ear
B. Middle ear
C. Cochlear nuclei
D. Medial geniculate body

23. The Helmoltz theory of color vision states that:

A. There are three kinds of cones in the retina responding to three primary colors
B. There are two kinds of cones called dominators and modulators
C. There is only one kind of cone and color is recognized only in area 17
D. There are seven types of cones responding to the seven colors of the spectrum

24. Pacinian corpuscles are the major receptors for:

A. Pain
B. Touch
C. Pressure
D. Temperature

25. Cold (Shivering) is regulated by:

A. Ant. hypothalamus
B. Post. hypothalamus
C. Thalamus
D. Pons

26. The cones in the eye are:

A. Not responsible for colour vision
B. More sensitive to light than the rods
C. Associated with higher visual acuity than the rods
D. Dependent on Vitamin A for their function

27. Meissner's corpuscles are believed to be sensitive to:

A. pH of interstitial fluid
B. Histamine
C. Change of temperature
D. Mechanical deformation

28. The receptors in semicircular canals respond to:

A. Linear acceleration
B. Angular acceleration
C. Both linear and angular acceleration
D. None of the above

29. Raised ECF K^+ levels seen in:

A. Endolymph
B. Ectolymph
C. Aqueous humour
D. Vitreous humour

30. **Site where endolymph is seen:**
    A. Scala vestibule
    B. Scala media
    C. Helicotrema
    D. All of the above

31. **Taste buds are:**
    A. Surface epithelial cells
    B. Specialised nerve endings
    C. Modified epithelial cells
    D. Chemoreceptors

32. **Which type of cone is it that has a peak absorbancy at a light wavelengths of 430 millimicrons?**
    A. Red cones B. Green cones
    C. Blue cones D. All of the above

33. **Receptors for touch is:**
    A. Meissner's
    B. Merkel's disc
    C. Free nerve terminal
    D. All of the above

34. **Normally body temperature can be raised by:**
    A. Androgens
    B. Gonadotropins
    C. Oestrogen
    D. Progesterone

35. **Kinesthetic sensations are detected mainly by what type of receptors?**
    A. Muscle spindles
    B. Golgi tendon apparatus
    C. Skin receptors
    D. Joint receptors

36. **Which of the following is wrong?**
    A. In the refracting eye, cornea causes more refraction than lens
    B. Fovea lies on the temporal side of the optic disc
    C. Cones are the more sensitive to light than rods
    D. Squint may result due to damage to internal capsule

37. **Rhodopsin is most sensitive and least sensitive to:**
    A. Violet light, red light
    B. Red light, violet light
    C. Green light, red light
    D. Blue light, green light

38. **The semicircular canals contain hair cells which are stimulated by:**
    A. Movement of perilymph
    B. Linear acceleration
    C. Cessation of rotation
    D. Rotation at constant velocity

39. **The sound becomes painful above decibel of:**
    A. 70 B. 86
    C. 140 D. 160

40. **The approximate refractive index of aqueous humour and vitreous humour is:**
    A. 1.21 B. 1.33
    C. 1.43 D. 1.56

41. **For normal eye of an adult, near point is situated at:**
    A. 9 cm B. 14 cm
    C. 20 cm D. 25 cm

42. **The optical power of the eye is:**
    A. 25 Diopters
    B. 50 Diopters
    C. 66 Diopters
    D. 75 Diopters

43. **The visible range in electromagnetic spectrum for human eye is:**

A. 200-300 nm B. 310-340 nm
C. 370-740 nm D. 740-870 nm

44. **Ear is most sensitive to the frequency (Hz) of:**

A. 300-500
B. 1000-3000
C. 10000-20000
D. None of the above

45. **The portion of the vestibular system that is most important for preventing a person from suddenly falling. If he makes a sudden turn while moving forward is the:**

A. Saccule
B. Utricle
C. Cochlea duct
D. Semicircular canals

46. **Which of the following is not important in dark adaptation?**

A. Conversion of retinene into rhodopsin
B. Conversion of Vitamin A into retinene
C. The pupillary reflex
D. Conversion of retinene into lumirhodopsin

EXPLANATORY ANSWERS OF SPECIAL SENSES

1. **Ans. D:** The ability of the eye to focus an object at varying distances is called accommodation. It involves contraction of ciliary muscle, constriction of pupil and convergence of visual axis. The tension exerted by the suspensory ligament on the lens is reduced, as a result the elastic lens bulges forwards and its anterior surface increases. (AK Jain 1139)
2. **Ans. D:** Air conducts sound waves to vibrate tympanic membrane. Solid ear ossicles vibrate to transmit vibration from tympanic membrane to oval window. The scala media is filled with endolymph. (AK Jain 1099,1102)
3. **Ans. C:** In the oral stage of deglutition, contraction of the front part of the tongue presses the bolus against the hard palate, while a series of movements of the middle part push it to the back, forcing it past the anterior pillar of the "fauces" (palatoglossal folds) to the root of the tongue. (AK Jain 214)
4. **Ans. A:** Merkel's disc and Meissner's corpuscles are concerned with perception of touch. They are rapidly adapting receptors. This is why we do not feel our clothes once they are put on. Pacinian corpuscles are concerned with the perception of pressure. They are quickly adapting. This is why we do not feel seat pressure when sitting. (AK Jain 889, 890)
5. **Ans. B:** The nerve is refractory or non responsive to a second stimulus, applied in quick succession to an area immediately behind the area of depolarization. (AK Jain 38)
6. **Ans. D:** The dark adaptation consists of two components: fast and slow response. Fast response is due to dark adaptation of the cones. It occurs over a period of 4-5 minutes. Slow response occurs over a period of 25 minutes. It involves resynthesis of rhodopsin in rods. Due to this one finds it initially difficulty to see on entering a dimly lit room. (AK Jain 1149)
7. **Ans. B:** Bitter taste is produced by cations. Substances that taste bitter act via G-protein coupled receptors and phospholipase C to cause release of calcium from endoplasmic reticulum. (AK Jain 1096, 1097)
8. **Ans. C:** Itching like pain originates from stimulation of free nerve endings in the skin and the nerve pathway: C group of fibers. (AK Jain 930)
9. **Ans. B:** Bitter taste is produced by many chemical substances like quinine sulphate, strychnine hydrochloride, morphine, nicotine, caffeine, urea, phenylthiourea, magnesium sulphate. Bitter taste is produced by cations. Substances that taste bitter act via G-protein coupled receptors and phospholipase C to cause release of calcium from endoplasmic reticulum. Bitter taste becomes unpleasant beyond a small degree and is rejected. (AK Jain 1096, 1097)
10. **Ans. D:** Tensor tympani and stapedius muscle get reflexly activated by loud sounds and decreases the amplitude of sound vibrations of tympanic membrane thus protecting internal ear from loud sounds. Reaction time is 40 to 160 msec. Therefore a sudden loud sound causes sudden displacement of hair cells from tectorial membrane resulting in deafness. (AK Jain 1101, 1109)
11. **Ans. B:** Primary colours are red, blue and green. Wavelength of orange is 600 nm. Thomas Yong Helmoltz theory states by mixing three primary colours in different

proportions, any type of colour sensation is produced. (AK Jain 1146,1156)

12. **Ans. B:** Ruffini end organs are encapsulated expanded endings of A delta and unmyelinated C group of fibers concerned with perception of warmth and mechanoreceptors. These are found in dermis and are slowly adapting receptors. (AK Jain 890)
13. **Ans. B:** Stapes foot plate is attached to oval window by annular ligament. (AK Jain 1101)
14. **Ans. C:** Cones in the eye are concerned with ABC: Acuity, Brightness and colour vision. (AK Jain 1124)
15. **Ans. C:** Visual acuity is maximum at the fovea centralis where the cones are closely packed and each has a connection with a single ganglion cell. The periphery of retina has visual acuity of less than 1/30th of that of fovea. (AK Jain 1136)
16. **Ans. C:** Taste is perceived by taste buds, carried by sensory fibers to Nucleus Tractus of Solitarius. Then they relay to the posteroventral nucleus of the thalamus. The third order neuron end in inferior part of posterior central gyrus. (AK Jain 1095)
17. **Ans. C:** Tensor tympani and stapedius muscle get reflexly activated by loud sounds and decreases the amplitude of sound vibrations of tympanic membrane thus protecting internal ear from loud sounds. Reaction time is 40 to 160 msec. Therefore a sudden loud sound causes sudden displacement of hair cells from tectorial membrane resulting in deafness. (AK Jain 1101, 1109)
18. **Ans. A:** The crude touch sensations are carried by the ventral spinothalamic tract. The touch is of high threshold of excitement and is poorly localized. (AK Jain 922)
19. **Ans. A:** After removal of the lens the diopteric power of the eye is reduced by 16 D. Therefore the cornea is responsible for 43 D of refractive power of the eye. Normal eye has a refractory power of 59 D. (AK Jain 1136)
20. **Ans. E:** Blockage of Canal of Schlemm leads to an increase in intraocular pressure above 80 mm Hg so the eyeball on palpation feels as hard as stone. This condition is called glaucoma. Normal pressure is 13-18 mm Hg. (AK Jain 1123)
21. **Ans. A:** Anterior two thirds are supplied by lingual nerve which branches from chorda tympani nerve, posterior one third of the tongue run in glossopharyngeal nerve. Taste is perceived by taste buds, carried by sensory fibers to Nucleus Tractus of Solitarius. Then they relay to the posteroventral nucleus of the thalamus. The third order neuron end in inferior part of posterior central gyrus. (AK Jain 1095)
22. **Ans. B:** The ear ossicles move as one unit to magnify sound intensity 1.2 to 1.3 times and also helps increase the pressure in the middle ear by 17 times. This is referred as Impedence matching, i.e., an effective transfer of sound energy from air to a fluid medium. Due to otosclerosis in the aged the lever system of ossicles cause high build up of pressure in middle ear of sound and old tympanic muscles fail to protect the middle ear from high pitched sounds like the violin striking his teeth (Eustachian tube connects the pharynx area to the middle ear). (AK Jain 1108)
23. **Ans. A:** Primary colors are red, blue and green. Thomas Yong Helmoltz theory states by mixing three primary colours in different proportions, any type of colour sensation is produced. When the three cones are stimulated equally white colour is produced. (AK Jain 1146,1156)
24. **Ans. C:** Pacinian corpuscles are concerned with the perception of pressure. They are

quickly adapting. This is why we do not feel seat pressure when sitting. (AK Jain 889, 890)

25. **Ans. B:** The anterior hypothalamus is the centre for responses to rising temperature and the posterior hypothalamus the centre for responses to falling temperature or cold. Shivering is an involuntary response of skeletal muscles contraction and can increase muscle metabolism up to three times. (AK Jain 596)
26. **Ans. C:** Cones in the eye are concerned with ABC: Acuity, Brightness and Colour vision. (AK Jain 1124)
27. **Ans. D:** Meissner's corpuscles are concerned with perception of touch. They are rapidly adapting receptors. This is why we do not feel our clothes once they are put on. (AK Jain 889)
28. **Ans. B:** The semicircular canals detect angular acceleration during rotation of head in the three perpendicular axis. (AK Jain 970)
29. **Ans. A:** The semicircular canals contain endolymph. The K+ concentration in scala media endolymph is 138 mEq/L. Is composition is similar to ICF, high in K+, low in Na+. (AK Jain 966, 1113)
30. **Ans. B:** The semicircular canals contain endolymph. Scala media of internal ear also has endolymph. The scala vestibule and scala tympani have perilymph. (AK Jain 1112)
31. **Ans. C:** Taste is perceived by taste buds. Taste buds are oval clusters of cells in epithelial layer with a small opening on the surface that allows substances to reach the interior of the taste bud. (AK Jain 1094)
32. **Ans. C:** There are three types of cones, each possessing its own characteristic photosensitive substance. These receptors subserve colour vision and respond maximally to light at wavelength 430 nm (blue colour or cyanolabe), 535 nm (green or chlorolabe) and 575 nm (red or erythrolabe). (AK Jain 1148)
33. **Ans. D:** Merkel's disc and Meissner's corpuscles are concerned with perception of touch. They are rapidly adapting receptors. This is why we do not feel our clothes once they are put on. Naked nerve endings are concerned with the perception of pain and noxious stimulus. They can also convey sensations of touch and temperature. (AK Jain 889,890)
34. **Ans. D:** Progesterone is a thermogenic hormone. Recording the basal body temperature before passing urine in the morning is an index of time of ovulation. In the pre-ovulatory phase the oral BBT is 36.3 to 36.8 °C which increases by 0.3-0.5 °C after ovulation. (AK Jain 826)
35. **Ans. D:** Proprioception means the sense of the body's position in space and kinesthesia refers to the sensation with joint movement. The major receptors are joint receptors. These are pacinian corpuscles, ruffini's end organs and golgi tendon organs which are situated in ligaments of the joints. They are quickly adapting receptors and form the endings of afferent nerves of group I fibers. (AK Jain 922,890)
36. **Ans. C:** Rhodopsin the pigment for rods is bleached by light. Rhodopsin the cone pigment is maximum sensitive at about 560 nm for greenish yellow light. (AK Jain 1147, 1148)
37. **Ans. C:** The maximum sensitivity of scotopic vision is approx. 500 nm, i.e., for bluish green light. This shows that red colour 650-700 nm is not at all sensitive to dim light. Thus in dim light, if blue and red colours need to be compared, blue can be made out easily. (AK Jain 1147)

38. **Ans. C:** The tops of the hair cells in the organ of corti are held rigid by the reticular lamina and their cilia are embedded in the tectorial membrane. The hair cells processes bend whenever there is a sharp motion or stoppage of motion between two stiff structures, the tectorial membrane and reticular lamina. This results in generation of action potential in the auditory nerve. (AK Jain 1109)

39. **Ans. C:** Painful and damaging sounds are at 140 dB. The intensity of sound at the maximum of the scale is actually 10^{14} times that required for hearing. Normal conversation is at 60 dB. Zero dB is standard or reference sound. (AK Jain 1107)

40. **Ans. C:** The refractive index or velocity of light in air/velocity of air in that substance is 1.37 in cornea, 1.33 in aqueous humour, 1.34 in vitreous humor and 1.42 for crystalline lens. For practical purposes the cornea and humors have same refractive index for practical purposes with refraction occurring at cornea and lens. (AK Jain 1135)

41. **Ans. D:** Near point of eye is at that point where the object can be seen clearly, with maximum accommodation of the lens. It is 25 cm. The near point recedes or moves away slowly as the age progresses due to loss of elasticity of the lens. (AK Jain 1141)

42. **Ans. C:** After removal of the lens the diopteric power of the eye is reduced by 16 D. Therefore the cornea is responsible for 43 D of refractive power of the eye. Normal eye has a refractory power of 59 D. (AK Jain 1136)

43. **Ans. C:** The eye responds to light of wavelengths between 400 nm and 750 nm called visibility or sensitivity range of vision. Below 400 nm or ultraviolet gets absorbed by choroids. Above 450 nm or infrared get absorbed by cornea. (AK Jain 1146)

44. **Ans. B:** Human ear can perceive pitch of sound between 16-20,000 cycles per sec or Hertz. It is maximally sensitive to pitch variations in the 1000-3000 Hz range. (AK Jain 1107)

45. **Ans. D:** The semicircular canals detect angular acceleration (while making a turn) during rotation of head in the three perpendicular axis. Saccule and Utricle provide information about linear acceleration and change in position relative to the force of gravity, i.e., vertical and horizontal acceleration respectively. (AK Jain 970)

46. **Ans. D:** Dark adaptation causes mydriasis or dilatation of pupils, change over of photoreceptor function from cones to rods, resynthesis of rhodopsin (from retinene, which is formed from Vitamn A1). Conversion of retinene into lumirhodopsin occurs in the light as the rods are bleached (turned white from visual purple). (AK Jain 1149)

CHAPTER 3

Cardiovascular System (CVS)

What is important in CVS?

ECG, Cardiac Output, Cardiac Cycle, Venous Return and Their Regulation, Coronary Circulation, Haemodynamics of Blood Flow (Especially to Heart, Lungs, Kidney etc), Dynamics of Shock

1. **The basis of Korotkow's sound is stated to be:**
   A. AV valve closure
   B. Aortic valve closure
   C. Arterial expansion
   D. Arterial turbulence

2. **Opening of aortic valves is initiated when:**
   A. Ventricular pressure exceeds aortic pressure
   B. Ventricles contract
   C. Ventricles relax
   D. Aortic contracts

3. **Essential hypertension is generally associated with an early increase in:**
   A. Oxygen use B. Coronary flow
   C. Cardiac work D. Cardiac output

4. **A hypertrophied ventricle will depolarize:**
   A. More rapidly than other ventricle
   B. Shift the electrical to involved side
   C. Before the other ventricle
   D. None of the above

5. **Changes in mean electrical axis of the ventricles may be caused by:**
   A. Muscular necrosis
   B. Bundle branch block
   C. Change in body position
   D. Hypertrophy of one ventricle
   E. All of the above

6. **Pulse pressure in a particular vessel is determined chiefly by:**
   A. Distance from heart
   B. Frictional characteristics of lumen
   C. Distensibility
   D. Cross-sectional area

7. **Sympathetic stimulation of heart causes:**
   A. Increased coronary flow
   B. Increased excitability of heart
   C. Increased force of myocardial contraction
   D. All of the above

8. **Parasympathetic stimulation of heart causes:**
   A. Decreased rate of S.A. node

B. Increased excitability of A-V junctional fibers
C. Prevents ventricular contraction
D. None of the above

9. Increased pressure within carotid sinus produces:

A. Reflex increase in venous pressure
B. Reflex hyperpnoea
C. Reflex bradycardia
D. Increase in heart rate

10. What is not true of "a" wave of venous pulsations in neck?

A. Exaggerated in tricuspid stenosis
B. Abolished in atrial fibrillation
C. Occurs just after in carotid artery
D. Exaggerated in complete heart block when P wave falls between QRS and T waves

11. In man cardiac cycle duration (sec) is:

A. 0.4 B. 0.8
C. 1 D. 1.6

12. Blood flow through left coronary artery:

A. Regulated by sympathetic vasodilator nerves
B. Increases when myocardial hypoxia
C. Greatest during early systole
D. Decrease in reflex response to fall in blood pressure

13. All is true for veins, except:

A. Innervated by sympathetic vasodilator nerves
B. Contain major part of blood volume
C. Respond to an increase in intraluminal pressure by constriction
D. Receive nutrition through vasa vasorum which arises from veins

14. Ventricular filling:

A. Produces third heart sound in some healthy persons
B. Depends mainly on contraction of atria
C. Begins during isometric ventricular relaxation
D. Will not occur unless atrial pressure is higher than atmospheric pressure

15. Sympathetic vasoconstrictor tone is diminished in response to increased activity of:

A. Carotid body chemoreceptors
B. Carotid sinus pressoreceptors
C. Pain receptors
D. Medullary chemoreceptors

16. When pacemaker is another area of heart, it denotes:

A. Wrong with conducting tissue
B. Wrong with SA node
C. Wrong with neural controlling system
D. None of the above

17. Dicrotic notch in aortic pressure curve is:

A. Magnified by aortic regurgitation
B. Absent in arteriosclerosis
C. Of no diagnostic value
D. Coincident with 2nd heart sound

18. Absolute refractory period of heart:

A. Heart is in diastole
B. Unresponsive to neural stimuli
C. No action potential from another part of heart will reexcite the heart muscle
D. None of the above

19. The law relating distending pressure and tension in a blood vessels wall is called:

A. Frank Starling law
B. Einthoven's law
C. Law of Laplace
D. Mary's law

20. Vascular distensibility is least for the following vascular segment:

A. Pulmonary artery B. Systemic artery
C. Systemic vein D. Pulmonary vein

21. Turbulant blood flow is produced by:

A. Decreased velocity of circulation
B. Decreased cardiac output
C. Decreased haematocrit
D. All of the above

22. Pulse pressure is lowest in:

A. Capillaries B. Arterioles
C. Radial artery D. Femoral artery

23. Oncotic pressure is measured by:

A. Osmal B. Arterioles
C. Radial artery D. Femoral artery

24. Following are increased during exercise except:

A. Cardiac output
B. Venous return
C. Coronary blood flow
D. Peripheral vascular resistance

25. To estimate cardiac output by dye-dilution technique, dye concentration is measured in:

A. Sample from peripheral artery
B. Sample from right atrium
C. Sample from aorta
D. Sample from pulmonary artery continously

26. What best characterises the sinusoids?

A. Have smaller diameter than lymph capillaries
B. Are not found in skeletal muscles
C. Have a continuous endothelial lining
D. Have a continuous basement membrane

27. Bhopal gas tragedy is caused by Methyl iso cyanate that causes J reflex. Which Indian scientist did single nerve studies to discover this reflex?

A. AS Paintal B. JC Bose
C. GK Chinnha D. BK Anand

28. Causes of hypoxic hypoxia include all except:

A. Kyphoscoliosis
B. Emphysema
C. Pulmonary fibrosis
D. Carbon monoxide poisoning

29. The most common form of hypoxia is:

A. Hypoxia B. Stagnant
C. Anemic D. Histitoxic

30. Hemoglobin has .... Times affinity for carbon monoxide than oxygen.

A. 50 B. 100
C. 210 D. 320

31. Carbon monoxide reacts with hemoglobin in form of:

A. Carboxy hemoglobin
B. Reduced hemoglobin
C. Cyanohemoglobin
D. Any of the above

32. Administration of oxygen rich gas mixtures is of value in all except:

A. Histitoxic hypoxia
B. Stagnant hypoxia
C. Anemic hypoxia
D. Hypoxic hypoxia

33. Which of the following is most fatal complications of increased barometric pressure?

A. Oxygen toxicity
B. Nitrogen narcosis
C. Air embolism
D. Decompensation sickness

34. The normal plasma oncotic pressure is:

A. 10 mm Hg B. 15 mm Hg
C. 20 mm Hg D. 30 mm Hg

35. The prime regulator of blood flow through exercising muscles is:

A. Venous tone
B. Sympathetic control
C. Vasodilator metabolites
D. Parasympathetic control

36. Blood pressure is not reliable in:

A. Coarctation of aorta
B. Pulmonary stenosis
C. Atrial fibrillation
D. Polyarteritis nodosa

37. Blood flow in ml/100 g min is maximum in:

A. Kidneys B. Liver
C. Heart D. Skin

38. After liver and kidneys, the blood flow is maximum in:

A. Brain
B. Skeletal muscle
C. Skin
D. Heart muscle

39. Major part of total peripheral resistance:

A. Medium and small arteries
B. Venules
C. Capillaries
D. Arterioles

40. Blood flow reaching the liver via portal versus hepatic artery is:

A. 2 : 1 B. 3 : 1
C. 4 : 1 D. 6 : 1

41. Hepatic blood flow is:

A. 500 ml/min B. 800 ml/min
C. 1200 ml/min D. 1500 ml/min

42. Heart receives about:

A. 1% cardiac output
B. 2% of cardiac output
C. 5% cardiac output
D. 10% cardiac output

43. Which of the following is true about composition of venous blood?

	PO_2 (mm Hg)	PCO_2 (mm Hg)	Hb (saturated %)
A.	95	40	75
B.	40	40	75
C.	40	46	75
D.	46	40	75

EXPLANATORY ANSWERS OF CVS

1. **Ans. D:** Korotkoff's sound is due to arterial turbulence. It is described as tapping, banging, muffling and disappearance. (AK Jain 363)
2. **Ans. A:** Opening of valves is a slowly developing process and does not produce any noise. When the pressure in the LV exceed the pressure in the aorta (80 mm Hg) and the pressure in the pulmonary artery (10 to 12 mm Hg), opening of semilunar occur. (AK Jain 298)
3. **Ans. C:** Essential or primary hypertension is defined as arterial BP >150/90 mm Hg. Cardiac output (SV, HR) and viscosity of the blood is normal, increased PR due to sympathetic overactivity or influence of Angiotensin, catecholamines cause increase in cardiac work. (AK Jain 416)
4. **Ans. B:** In left ventricular hypertrophy abnormal left axis deviation (LAD) of mean QRS vector left of -30 occurs. In right ventricular hypertrophy RAD right of + 110° is present. (AK Jain 310)
5. **Ans. E:** Abnormal axis deviation is caused by bundle branch bloc, ventricular hypertrophy and myocardial infarction. (AK Jain 310)
6. **Ans. C:** In advancing age due to loss in elasticity of blood vessels, stretching decreases which results in increased pressure during systole with normal diastolic blood pressure (systolic hypertension). The blood vessels behave like a rigid tube. It is characterized by high pulse pressure. Pulse pressure is determined by elasticity of vessel wall that varies inversely with total peripheral resistance. (AK Jain 363)
7. **Ans. D:** Sympathetic stimulation (T1-T5) increases heart rate (chronotropic action), increases speed and force of myocardium contraction (ionotropic), increases conductivity in conducting tissue (positive chronotropic) and increases excitability of heart (positive bathmotropic). (AK Jain 338)
8. **Ans. A:** Parasympathetic supply decrease rate of impulse generation by SAN causing heart rate to decrease (negative chronotropic). (AK Jain 340)
9. **Ans. C:** Due to pressure on carotid sinus produced by tight collar, marked bradycadia and hypotension is produced. (AK Jain 413)
10. **Ans. C:** There is no valve at junction of superior vena cava (SVC) and right atrium (RA) therefore right atrial pressure changes are transmitted to the jugular vein in the neck. "a" wave is due to atrial systole. Some blood regurgitates into the great veins when atria contracts, even though the orifices of IVC and SVC are constricted. In addition veins inflow stops, causing rise in venous pressure, contributing to the "a" wave. (AK Jain 301)
11. **Ans. B:** Cardiac cycle normal duration is 0.8 sec at heart rate of 75/min. Ventricular systole 0.3 sec, ventricular diastole 0.5 sec, atrial systole 0.1 sec and atrial diastole 0.7 sec. (AK Jain 297)
12. **Ans. B:** Myocardial hypoxia causes formation of adenosine, a vasodilator metabolite that increases Coronary blood flow (phenomenon called reactive hyperemia). (AK Jain 383)
13. **Ans. D:** Veins are capacitance vessels, which simply change their luminal shape to accommodate large volume of blood without much increase in transmural pressure. (AK Jain 326)

14. **Ans. A:** The third heart sounds (HS_3) is due to vibrations of cardiac walls produced by rapid filling phase of the ventricles during ventricular diastole proper. It has low intensity and is 0.1 sec duration. (AK Jain 301)

15. **Ans. B:** Reduction of sympathetic constrictor tone occurs in condition of flushed skin of stress, via hypothalamus, vasodilation of skeletal muscle, viscera, skin and blood vessels through baroreceptors. (AK Jain 340)

16. **Ans. B:** SAN is called the cardiac pacemaker and its rate of discharge normally determines the rate at which the heart beats. (AK Jain 294)

17. **Ans. D:** During protodiastole the arterial pressure exceeds that in the ventricles and results in sharp closure of semilunar valves causing sharp (HS_2) or dicrotic notch. (AK Jain 300)

18. **Ans. C:** Cardiac muscle is refractory, i.e., non-responsive to restimulation during most part of action potential. Normal refractory period (ARP) is 180-200 msec and relative refractory period (RRP) is upto 50 msec. (AK Jain 180)

19. **Ans. C:** Law of Laplace states that the distending pressure (P) in a distensible hollow object is equal to the tension in the wall (T) divided by the radius of curvature (R). P=2T/R. (AK Jain 332)

20. **Ans. B:** Skin and skeletal muscles blood vessels represents by far the most important site of peripheral resistance and offer maximum respiration to blood flow. (AK Jain 325)

21. **Ans. C:** Turbulent blood flow is given by Reynold's number (Re)=Vρd/n where V is velocity of flow in cm/sec, ρ density of density of blood equal to 1, d is the diameter of blood vessel, n is viscosity of blood in poise. Turbulence develops when Re exceeds 2000. Viscosity is directly proportional to haematocrit, i.e., packed cell volume, concentration of plasma protein, diameter of vessel wall because of plasma skimming. Viscosity decreases when vessel wall diameter falls below 300 μm due to secretion of mucpolysaccharide. Re > 3000 turbulence is present, < 2000 no turbulence is present. (AK Jain 331)

22. **Ans. A:** Pulse pressure is the difference between systolic and diastolic pressure (50 mm Hg). Pressure falls very slightly in large and medium sized arteries but rapidly in small arteries and arteroles. The pulse pressure decline rapidly to 5 mm at the end of arterioles. (Ganong 22nd edition 587)

23. **Ans. A:** Colloidal osmotic pressure due to plasma colloids is called oncotic pressure. (AK Jain 15)

24. **Ans. D:** Sympathetic vasodilator nerve dilate the arterioles only. Therefore during exercise vascular peripheral resistance of muscle blood vessels decrease allowing more blood supply. (AK Jain 400)

25. **Ans. A:** Dye is injected into vein, it passes though the heart, then pulmonary circulation and finally will be evenly distributed in blood stream. Hence sample is taken from peripheral artery. (AK Jain 301)

26. **Ans. B:** Sinusoids are discontinuous capillaries , possess a thin endothelial layer with large gaps between individual cells. Therefore, allow easy exchange of large protein molecules. Bone marrow, liver and spleen are the sites. (AK Jain 326)

27. **Ans. A:** J receptors are sensitive to the content of interstitial fluid between the capillary endothelium and alveolar epithelium. They respond to pulmonary congestion, pulmonary embolisation, pulmonary oedema and inhaling of strong

irritants/chemicals. Tachypnoea is rapid shallow respiration. J receptors have a physiological role in severe exercise, cause an increase in interstitial fluid in the lungs. J receptors get stimulated, inhibiting spinal stretch reflex and thus limit the power of contraction of skeletal muscle. (AK Jain 471)

28. **Ans. D:** CO poisoning is a form of anemic hypoxia, as Carboxy hemoglobin is formed preventing hemoglobin to combine with oxygen. (AK Jain 487)
29. **Ans. A:** The most common form of hypoxia is hypoxic hypoxia. At tissue level, the oxygen utilization is 5 ml % in normal as well as hpoxic hypoxia (high altitude). (AK Jain 486)
30. **Ans. C:** Haemoglobin has 250 times affinities for CO. (AK Jain 57)
31. **Ans. A:** Carbon monoxide reacts with hemoglobin in the form of carboxy hemoglobin. (AK Jain 57)
32. **Ans. A:** Administration of oxygen gas mixtures is of no value in histotoxic hypoxia. Histotoxic hypoxia: Hypoxia in which the amount of oxygen delivered to the tissue cells is adequate but because of the action of a toxic agent the tissue cells cannot make use of the oxygen supplied to them. (AK Jain 489)
33. **Ans. C:** Entry of air into the blood circulation may cause death. (A K Jain 501)
34. **Ans. D:** Colloidal osmotic pressure due to plasma colloids means same as that of oncotic pressure. The normal oncotic pressure is 25 mm Hg or 30 mm Hg. (AK Jain 53)
35. **Ans. C:** The prime regulator of blood flow through exercising muscle is vasodilator metabolites. (AK Jain 325)
36. **Ans. C:** Blood pressure is not reliable in atrial fibrillation. Excitation waves causes irregular contractions. So BP is also not regular. (AK Jain 315)
37. **Ans. A:** Normally renal blood flow is 1.2 to 1.3 L/min, i.e., 300-400 ml/100 gm/min. Coronary blood flow is 60 to 80 ml/100 gm/min, Brain 55 ml/100 gm/min, skeletal muscle 3-4 ml/100 gm/min. (AK Jain 525)
38. **Ans. B:** After liver (1300 ml) and kidneys (1200 ml) the blood flow is maximum in skeletal muscle (1000 ml). (AK Jain 325)
39. **Ans. D:** Resistance vessels are arterioles. (AK Jain 324)
40. **Ans. A:** Blood flow (ml/min) reaching the liver via portal versus hepatic artery is 1200: 300=4:1. (AK Jain 245)
41. **Ans. A:** Hepatic artery is 1500 ml/min. 300 ml/min from hepatic artery, 1200 ml/min from portal venous supply. (AK Jain 245)
42. **Ans. C:** Heart receives about 5% of cardiac output. Blood flow to the heart=250 ml/min. Cardiac output = 5000 ml/min (approx). Therefore % of cardiac output going to heart (250/5000) × 100 = 5%. (AK Jain 355)
43. **Ans. C:** PO_2 (mm of Hg) is 40 and PCO_2 is 46. (AK Jain 463)

CHAPTER 4

Endocrinology

Important Topics:

Pituitary, Thyroid, Pancreas, Parathyroid, Sexual Function

1. **All the following pituitary hormones are derived from basophilic and acidophilic cells except:**
   A. GH B. ACTH
   C. PIH D. FSH

2. **All of the following are true insulin except:**
   A. Glucose is absorbed from renal tubules'
   B. Short polypeptide with C-chain
   C. Proinsulin is coiled and cross linked by disulfide bonds
   D. Proinsulin is inactive

3. **Cortisol:**
   A. Secretion increases following injury
   B. Favours protein synthesis
   C. Enhances effects of antigen-antibody reactions
   D. Tends to lower blood pressure

4. **Aldosteronism is associated with:**
   A. Oedema
   B. Retention of sodium
   C. Hypotension
   D. Retention of potassium

5. **Calcitonin is responsible for:**
   A. Increasing the plasma calcium level
   B. Decreasing the calcium level
   C. Increasing the parathormone level
   D. Decreasing thyroxine level

6. **Regarding Myxoedema the following are true except:**
   A. Swollen, Oedematous look of the face
   B. Impotency, amenorrhoea etc
   C. BMR increased by 30-40%
   D. Dullness, loss of memory

7. **The following features are found in hyperthyroidism except:**
   A. Enlarged thyroid
   B. Exophthalmos
   C. Decreased body weight
   D. Decreased BMR

8. **Regarding parathyroid the following statements are true except:**

A. It regulates Ca and P metabolism
B. Controls the balance of inorganic ions in blood
C. It is not essential for life
D. Its cellular effects are mediated through cAMP

9. **In Cushing syndrome the following features are found except:**
A. Rapidly increasing adiposity
B. Polycythemia
C. Hypotension
D. Impotence with atrophy of testis

10. **Progesterone is secreted by the following except:**
A. Corpus luteum B. Placenta
C. Adrenal cortex D. Testis

11. **Epinephrine predominantly causes:**
A. Glycogenolysis
B. Gluconeogenesis
C. Glycolysis
D. Glycogen storage

12. **Estrogens in the postmenopausal period is metabolized mostly into:**
A. Estriol
B. Estrone
C. Estradiol
D. Androstenedione

13. **FSH is secreted by:**
A. Chromophobes
B. Acidophils
C. Basophils
D. Theca internal cells

14. **Sertoli cells secrete:**
A. Testosterone
B. Androstenedione
C. PGE_2
D. Esrtrogens

15. **In the absence of ADH (Anti-diuretic Hormone):**
A. There would not be any absorption in renal tubules
B. Facultative water absorption is deficient
C. Facultative water absorption is increased
D. Obligatory water absorption is increased

16. **TSH is secreted at a higher rate:**
A. After removal of one lobe of thyroid
B. In warm adapted than in cold adapted persons
C. When BMR falls
D. During physical injury and emotional stress

17. **The likelihood of developing tetany is increased when:**
A. Plasma HCO_3 rises
B. Plasma magnesium rises
C. Respiratory failure develops
D. Anterior pituitary removed

18. **Growth hormone secretion is increased in normal person in all of the following except:**
A. Exercise
B. Hyperglycemia
C. Infusion of Levodopa
D. Infusion of Arginine

19. **A patient with a secreting tumour of adrenal medulla (phaeochromocytoma) typically has:**
A. Raised blood pressure transient or constant

B. A fine tremor of extended hand
C. Lowering of blood pressure when alpha adrenoceptor
D. Increase in BMR
E. All of the above

20. Deficient adrenal function leads to rise in blood:

A. Sodium B. Glucose
C. Pressure D. Potassium

21. Steroids are synthesized by:

A. Smooth ER B. Rough ER
C. Mitochondria D. Lysososmes

22. Insulin promotes transport of glucose in which of these?

A. Adipose tissue B. RBC
C. Muscles D. Hepatocytes

23. Following are changes seen in SIADH except:

A. Low plasma osmolality
B. Low urine osmolality
C. Hyponatremia
D. Edema

24. Which neurotransmitter controls secretion of Prolactin?

A. Dopamine B. Serotonin
C. Somatostatin D. GABA

25. Increase in Insulin receptors is seen in:

A. Acromegaly B. Starvation
C. Obesity D. Diabetes

26. Menopausal hot flushes is due to:

A. FSH surge
B. LH surge
C. Decreased estrogen
D. Decreased progesterone

27. Which of the following is not caused by estrogen?

A. Decrease in Serum alkaline phosphatase
B. Increase Blood sugar
C. Increase Folate level
D. Increase HDL

28. Estrogens acts on:

A. Cell membrane
B. Nucleus
C. Mitochondria
D. Cytoplasmic receptor

29. Following are true of insulin except:

A. Glycopeptide
B. Secreted by beta cells
C. Causes lipogenesis
D. Promotes glycogenesis

30. Anabolic action on proteins is mediates by:

A. Growth hormone B. Insulin
C. ACTH D. Testosterone

31. Transection of the Pituitary stalk leads to increase in:

A. Growth Hormone B. TSH
C. Prolactin D. ACTH

32. Enzyme involved in acetylcholine synthesis is:

A. Choline acetyl transferase
B. Choline esterase
C. Pseudocholinesterase
D. Glycine

33. What determines whether norepinephrine circulating in the body fluids will be excitatory or inhibitory in a particular organ?

A. The nature of the receptor in the cells of the oxygen
B. The intensity of nerve stimulation
C. The chemical changes that occur in the norepinephrine before it excites the cells
D. The position on the cells where norepinephrine is secreted by the nerve endings

34. Alpha and beta types of receptors are used to explain pharmacological actions of:

A. Cholinergic B. Adrenergic
C. Muscarinic D. Nicotinic

35. Hormone secreted by hypothalamus is:

A. Somatostatin B. Somataotropin
C. Gonadotropin D. Luteotrophin

36. Following are local hormone except:

A. Insulin B. Heparin
C. Bradykinin D. Acetylcholine

37. The hormone with the shortest half life in the blood stream in the following list is:

A. Epinephrine B. Acetylcholine
C. Insulin D. T_3

38. Which of the following hormones is not secreted by the adenohypohysis?

A. ADH B. ACTH
C. TSH D. FSH

39. The thyroid hormone stored in the lumen of follicles is in the form of:

A. Free T_3
B. Free T_4
C. Attached to thyroglobulin
D. Attached to thyroid binding globulin

40. Hyperglycemia is associated with:

A. Decreased Insulin secretion
B. Increase Glucagon secretion
C. Increase Insulin and Glucagon secretion
D. A and B

41. Hyperthyroidism is associated with:

A. Positive nitrogen balance
B. A decreased urinary excretion of calcium
C. A rise in level of plasma protein which binds thyroxine
D. Certain feature due to excessive beta adrenergic stimulation

42. Thyroxine causes following except:

A. Increased BMR
B. Increased cholesterol
C. Increased beta-1 receptors
D. Increased heat production

43. Menopause is caused due to:

A. Endometrium becomes insensitive to oestrogen and progesterone
B. Ovary does not produce estrogen and progesterone
C. Pituitary
D. Hypothalamus

44. Aldosterone secretion is regulated by following except:

A. ACTH B. Calcium
C. Blood volume D. Potassium

45. Which of the following is not true about calcium metabolism?

A. Phytates in diet increase absorption
B. Dihydroxycholecalciferol increases absorption

C. High protein diet increase absorption
D. 40% of total calcium is in ionized form

46. Production of aldosterone under normal conditions will be influenced by all except:

A. Blood sodium level
B. Blood angiotensin level
C. Crystalloid osmotic pattern of blood
D. ACTH

47. Activation of rennin-angiotensin mechanism result in the following except:

A. Aldosterone secretion
B. Increased arteriolar tone
C. Decrease in renal sodium excretion
D. Decrease in blood volume

48. Calcium metabolism is mainly dependent on:

A. Calcitonin
B. Parathormone
C. Thyroxine
D. Growth Hormone

49. Which of the following arterioles is least sensitive to epinephrine?

A. Skeletal muscle arteriole
B. Cerebral arteriole
C. Cutaneous arteriole
D. Afferent renal arteriole

50. Which of the following G Protein is associated with receptors for norepinephrine?

A. Gt1 B. Gi1
C. Gt2 D. Go

51. The following hormones increase the level of intracellular cAMP except:

A. Vasopressin
B. Glucagon
C. Estrogen
D. Somatostatin

52. Which of the following arterioles is least sensitive to epinephrine?

A. Skeletal muscle arteriole
B. Cerebral
C. Cutaneous
D. Afferent renal

53. Amino acid sequence of human insulin differs from porcine insulin in:

A. 1 amino acid
B. 3 amino acids
C. 5 amino acids
D. None of the above

54. Following are the effects of testosterone except:

A. Increased Haemopoiesis
B. Calcium retention
C. Increased total quantity of bone matrix
D. Increased BMR

55. Peak testosterone levels are seen at about:

A. 7-8 am B. 2 am
C. 7-8 pm D. 12 pm

56. In diabetic ketosis, there is a decreased metabolic breakdown of:

A. Fat B. Protein
C. Glucose D. Glycogen liver

57. The only hormone for which no stimulatory factor has been isolated is:

A. Growth hormone B. Gonadotrpin
C. Thyroxine D. Prolactin

58. Gluconeogenesis requires the action of:

A. Glucagons B. Insulin
C. Estradiol D. Calcitonin

59. Uterine contractility is increased by hormone:

A. Progesterone B. LH
C. FSH D. Oestrogen

60. In the testes, the cells that secrete testosterone are:

A. Germinal epithelium
B. Leydig cells
C. Sertoli cells
D. Sperm cells

61. Which of the following does not act at receptors?

A. TRH B. Thyroxine
C. Insulin D. Epinephrine

62. Which of the following statements is not correct? Release of acetylcholine at the neuromuscular junction:

A. Produces an end-plate potential
B. Increase sodium movement into the muscle cell
C. Always causes the muscle fiber to contract
D. Is followed by rapid destruction of acetylcholine

63. Somatostatin inhibits all except:

A. GH B. ACTH
C. TSH D. Prolactin

64. Experimental diabetes is caused by:

A. Alloxan
B. PGE_2
C. Radioactive yttrium
D. Gold chloride

65. Melatonin is secreted by:

A. Hypothalamus B. Adrenal cortex
C. Pineal gland D. Melanocytes

66. Which of the following decreases insulin secretion?

A. Growth hormone
B. Epinephrine
C. Glucocorticoids
D. Glucose

67. The secretion of aldosterone is caused by:

A. Angiotensin B. ACTH
C. Epinephrine D. Insulin

Match the following:

A. Cortisol
B. Androgen
C. Aldosterone
D. Norepinephrine

68. Zona glomerulosa

69. Zona reticularis

70. Zona fasciculate

71. Adrenal medulla

72. Hormones secreted by anterior pituitary is/are:

A. GH B. Prolactin
C. TSH D. All

73. Position of estradiol/OH is at:

A. C3 and C17 B. C 4 and C18
C. C 5 and C19 D. C 6 and C20

74. FSH and ICSH are secreted by:

A. Adenohypophysis
B. Hypothalamus
C. Ovaries
D. Placenta

75. **Metyrapone is useful in congenital hyperplasia because it inhibits:**
A. 17-alpha hydroxylase
B. 21-alpha hydroxylase
C. 11-beta hydroxylase
D. Desmolase

76. **Precursor of testosterone is:**
A. Methyltestosterone
B. Pregnanaolone
C. Aldosterone
D. Cortisone

77. **Function of Leutinising hormone is:**
A. Follicle maturation and ovulation
B. Milk secretion
C. Causes progesterone secretion during ovulation
D. Maintain placenta

78. **Cyclic AMP serves as second messenger in the secretion of all except:**
A. FSH B. Estrogen
C. Glucagon D. Epinephrine

79. **Pain producing substance is:**
A. Serotonin B. Substance P
C. Histamine D. Acetylcholine

80. **Which of the following is an endocrine organ?**
A. Lamina dura B. Small intestine
C. Ciliary body D. Breast

81. **True about gastrin is:**
A. A peptide hormone
B. An analogue of Pentagastrin which decreases secretion of HCl
C. Secreted with HCl from parietal cells
D. Increased in Zollinger-Ellison syndrome

82. **If there is a decrease in extracelluar fluid volume, the body may respond by increasing the secretion of:**
A. Epinephrine
B. Aldosterone
C. Epinephrine and aldosterone
D. Epinephrine, aldosterone and ADH

83. **Increased release of aldosterone from adrenal cortex is not a feature in:**
A. Increased arterial pressure
B. Hyponatremia
C. Hyperkalemia
D. Epinephrine and Norepinephrine

84. **When a patient is treated with aldosterone antagonist there is likely to be a fall in:**
A. Urine volume
B. Plasma potassium level
C. Blood volume
D. Blood viscosity

85. **An animal deprived of its adrenal glands:**
A. Loses most of its reactions due to increased sympathetic activity because of the lack of circulating epinephrine
B. Can still develop tachycardia and sympathetic hypertension in response to exercise
C. Has a much greater rate of glycogenolysis
D. Usually is hyperglycemic during fasting periods

86. **Which of the following responses is not initiated by the stimulation of adrenergic sympathetic neurons?**
A. Hepatic glycogenolysis

B. Skeletal muscle vasoconstriction
C. Ventricular conduction time increase
D. Contraction of pyloric sphincter of stomach

87. Pheochromocytomas predominantly secrete:

A. Epinephrine B. Norepinephrine
C. 5-HT D. Renin

88. Islet cells of pancreas secrete all of the following except:

A. Somatostatin B. Gastrin
C. VIP D. Pancreozymin

89. The following is true about carbonic anhydrase except:

A. A protein with a molecular weight of 30,000
B. Contains an item of copper in each molecule
C. Inhibited by cyanide, azide and sulfide
D. Sulfonamides also inhibit this enzyme

90. The size and number of inclusions in the type II alveolar epithelial cells producing surfactant are increased by:

A. Growth hormone B. Androgens
C. Cortisol D. Insulin

91. Important effects of testosterone include all of the following except:

A. Formation of the fetal penis
B. Descent of the testes into scrotum
C. Increased muscle development
D. Initiation of ejaculation

92. The active form of Vitamin D is:

A. Calcitonin
B. 1,25 Dihydroxycholecalciferol
C. Parathyroid hormone
D. Cholecalciferol

93. Increased plasma parathyroid hormone concentration tends to increase all of the following except:

A. Number of active osteoclasts
B. Extracellular phosphate concentration
C. Absorption of calcium from the gastrointestinal tract
D. Absorption of calcium from the renal tubules

94. All of the following hormones mediate their major effects without actually entering the target cell except:

A. Cortisol B. Insulin
C. Growth hormone D. Glucagon

95. Growth hormone increases all of the following except:

A. Cortisol B. Insulin
C. Dopamine D. Glucagon

96. Cortisol can cause all of the following except:

A. Inflammation to be suppressed
B. Fat to be used for energy
C. Lysosomal membranes to become unstable
D. The blood glucose concentration to increase

97. Thyroid stimulating hormone stimulates thyroid function in many ways, but it does not increase:

A. Synthesis of thyroxine-binding globulin
B. Rate of synthesis of thyroglobulin
C. Iodine uptake from the blood
D. Iodination of tyrosine

98. Hormones secreted by the thyroid gland include:

A. Thyroxine
B. Triiodothyronine

C. Calcitonin

D. All of the above

99. Most potent vasopressor is:

A. Angiotensin II B. Renin

C. Aldosterone D. Endothelin

100. High plasma levels of thyroxine can lead to all of the following except:

A. Increased cardiac output

B. Increased plasma triglyceride concentration

C. Increased heart rate

D. Decreased body weight

101. Blockage of the hypothalamic-hypophyseal venous portal system would be expected to cause increased secretion of:

A. Growth hormone

B. Adrenocorticotropic hormone

C. Thyroid stimulating hormone

D. Prolactin

102. Levels of which of the following hormones are increased in postmenopausal women?

A. Estrogen B. FSH

C. Progesterone D. Cortisone

103. Most potent vasopressor is:

A. Angiotensin II B. Renin

C. Aldosterone D. Cortisol

104. Beta endorphins are found in high concentration in:

A. Substantia gelatinosa

B. Post pituitary

C. Spinal cord

D. Medulla

105. Which is not formed in tryptophan metabolism?

A. Melatonin B. Dopamine

C. Serotonin D. None of above

106. Secretion of estriol during pregnancy:

A. Is independent on both a viable fetus and a functioning placenta

B. Is largely produced by the maternal ovaries

C. Is not dependent on a viable fetus

D. Is lower than the secretion rate of estriol is non-pregnancy body

107. The hormone responsible for increased body temperature after ovulation is:

A. Progesterone B. LH

C. FSH D. Oestrogen

108. Which of the following does not have natriuretic actions?

A. Aldosterone

B. Natriuretic peptide

C. Angiotensin

D. Prednisolone

109. Function of acini in thyroid gland is synthesis of:

A. Thyroxine B. Tyrosine

C. Mucus D. TSH

110. Calcitonin is produced by:

A. Thyroid B. Parathyroid

C. Thymus D. Kidney

111. Overall regulating organ for neuro-endocrinal system is:

A. Hypothalamus

B. Pituitary

C. Reticuloendothelial

D. Pineal gland

112. After drinking a large amount of hypotonic fluid and after absorption of the fluid and after absorption of the

fluid from the gut into the blood, which of the following changes would you expect?

A. Increased secretion of antidiuretic hormone
B. A decrease in distal tubular permeability to water
C. A marked decrease in glomerular filtration rate
D. A marked increase in sodium excretion

113. Stimulation of both glucorticorticoid and mineralocorticoid secretion is seen with:

A. Anxiety
B. Exercise
C. Hyperkalemia
D. Low sodium diet

114. "C" cells are present in:

A. Thyroid
B. Adrenal
C. Parathyroid
D. Pituitary

115. Spontaneous hypoglycemia may be caused by:

A. Glucagonoma
B. Chronic pancreatitis
C. Cushing's syndrome
D. Hepatocellular carcinoma

116. In the female rat, selective neutralization of follicle-stimulating hormone with ant-FSH antibodies:

A. Increases estrogen and progesterone secretion by the corpus luteum
B. Prevents early uniting of the epiphyses
C. Prevents early follicular growth
D. Suppresses the secretion of hypothalamic releasing factors

117. The following substances cross blood brain barrier:

A. Insulin
B. Testosterone
C. Glucose
D. All of the above

118. Vitamin D deficiency leads to:

A. Decreased calcium absorption by renal tubules
B. Decreased calcium absorption by intestine
C. Increased phosphate excretion by renal tubules
D. None of the above

119. In which of the following organ, glucose uptake depends on insulin?

A. Renal epithelium
B. Heart
C. Brain
D. Intestinal epithelium

120. Which of the following statements about calcitonin is false?

A. It reduces the number and activity of osteoclasts
B. It reduces the renal tubular absorption of calcium
C. It reduces the renal tubular absorption of phosphate
D. When present in excess, it commonly causes tetany

121. Which of the following statements about androgen is false?

A. They are formed by seminiferous tubules of the testis
B. They are formed in greater quantities is foetal life (in the male foetus) than in childhood
C. Are secreted in small amounts in normal audit females
D. Their concentration in blood decreases after the age of 30 in men

122. Which of the following statements about thyroxine is false?

A. Its production requires the aminoacids tyrosine
B. Its effect is slower in onset and longer in duration than that of triiodothyronine (T3)
C. It increases cerebral metabolic oxygen consumption
D. It is essential for the production of erythrocytes

123. The principal estrogen found in the urine of pregnant women is:

A. Estriol B. Estrone
C. Beta-estradiol D. Pregnanediol

124. Cortisol increases the blood glucose concentration either directly or indirectly by:

A. Decreasing glucose uptake by the cells
B. Decreasing the rate of gluconeogenesis
C. Decreasing the rate of glucose utilization by the cells
D. Inhibiting hormone-sensitive lipase

125. Synthesis of testosterone is controlled by:

A. LH B. LHRH
C. FSH D. TSH

126. All of the following are the actions of glucocorticoids on blood cells except:

A. Decrease in number of Eosinophils
B. Decrease in the number of Basophils
C. Increase in the number of Lymphocytes
D. Increase in the number of neutrophils and platelets
E. Increase in the number of Red Blood cells

127. A cortisol deficient individual:

A. Has reduced resistance to stress
B. Has increased ability to mobilize stored triglyceride
C. Has reduced sensitivity to insulin
D. Shows all of these

128. Every nucleated cell has one of the following proteins which is involved in transmission of the message of many hormones called:

A. Calcium binding protein
B. Calmodulin
C. Apotransferrin
D. Apoceruloplasmin

129. The hormone which diminishes the excretion of magnesium is:

A. Anti-diuretic hormone
B. Parathormone
C. Growth hormone
D. Aldosterone

130. The prohormone produced by the theca interna of the ovary is:

A. 17- Ketosteroid
B. An estrogen
C. A dehydroepiandrosterone
D. All of these

131. Gonadal function is regulated by:

A. Anterior hypothalamus
B. Posterior hypothalamus
C. Anterior pituitary
D. Posterior pituitary

132. Level of T3 indicates:

A. Metabolic state
B. Thyroid state
C. Pituitary function state
D. Not important

133. Spermatogenic epithelium is maintained by:

A. Somatostatin B. TRH

C. FSH D. LH

134. Dopamine is inhibitor of:

A. Prolactin

B. Growth hormone

C. Oxytocin

D. Epinephrine

135. Actions of insulin are all except:

A. Glycolysis

B. Glycogenesis

C. Lipogenesis

D. Gluconeogenesis

136. Reverse T3 is:

A. Synthetic derivative

B. Isomerisation product of T4 active

C. Isomerisation product of T3 inactive

D. Reverse T4

137. Which of the following hormone acts by decreasing cAMP levels?

A. Epinephrine (Beta 1 receptors)

B. Dopamine (D2 receptors)

C. Glucagon

D. None of the above

138. Luteal phase of menstrual cycle is characterized by:

A. A variable length

B. Secretion of estrogen

C. Low basal body temperature

D. Secretion of progesterone

139. ACTH is most effective in stimulating the secretion of:

A. Hydrocortisone

B. Cortisone

C. Adrenal androgenic hormones

D. Aldosterone

140. On injecting concentrated NaCl solution into the carotid artery, there was increased production of ADH. The source of its secretion in the hypothalamus is in the:

A. Paraventricular nucleus

B. Supraoptic nucleus

C. Anterior nucleus

D. Ventromedial nucleus

141. Which is produced in Cushing's syndrome in excess?

A. Epinephrine

B. Norepinephrine

C. Cortisol

D. Dopamine

142. Thyroxine does not increase the metabolism in:

A. Heart B. Liver

C. Pituitary D. Kidney

143. Secretion of which of the following does not increase in night:

A. Growth Hormone B. ACTH

C. Insulin D. TSH

144. Which of the following feature is not seen in hypopituitary state?

A. Cachexia

B. Growth failure

C. Infertility

D. Increased sensitivity to insulin

145. Lack of which of the following hormone causes osteoporosis?

A. Oestrogen B. Progesterone

C. Thyroxine D. Testosterone

146. A person who is on starvation for 5 days. Glucose is given for GTT will cause the following except:

A. GH decrease
B. Decreased insulin
C. Increased cortisol
D. Increased insulin tolerance

147. FSH is produced by:

A. Chromophobes
B. Acidophils
C. Basophils
D. All of the above

148. Thyroxine is injected to rat causes all except:

A. Decrese Lipolysis
B. Increase oxygen consumption
C. Decrease BMR
D. Increase myocardial contractility

149. cAMP action mediates all except:

A. Glucagon   B. FSH
C. LH   D. Estrogen

150. Which of the following statements about progesterone is not true?

A. It stimulates the development of lobules and alveoli in the breast
B. It increases the excitability of myometrium
C. It is thermogenic
D. It can prevent ovulation in large doses
E. In large doses it produces natriuresis

151. The laboratory report shows values of gonadotropin and ovarian hormones of the blood sample taken on day 20 of the menstural cycle of a young woman. Whether her cycle was ovulatory or not may be validly assessed by the reported serum level of:

A. FSH   B. LH
C. Oestradiol   D. Progesterone

152. Even in the presence of vasopressin the greatest fraction of filtered water is reabsorbed in which part of the nephron?

A. Proximal tubule   B. Distal tubule
C. Loop of Henle   D. Collecting duct

153. The hormone associated with cold adaptation is:

A. Growth hormone
B. Thyroxine
C. Insulin
D. Melanocyte stimulating hormone

EXPLANATORY ANSWERS OF ENDOCRINOLOGY

1. **Ans. C:** 75% chromophils exists as Acidophils and Basophils. Acidophils stain red and are of two types: Somatotrophs secreting growth hormone and mammotrophs secreting prolactin. Basophils are of three types: Gonadotrophs secreting LH and FSH, Thyrotrophs secreting TSH and Corticotrophs secreting ACTH, β LPH. (AK Jain 667)

2. **Ans. A:** Glucose transport across the following cells does not require insulin:
   (a) Brain except ventromedial nucleus of hypothalamus.
   (b) Kidney tubules, GIT and RBC's.

   Thus brain cannot withstand hypoglycemia. In diabetic patients glucose absorption from Kidney tubules, GIT and RBC's remain unaffected. (AK Jain 767)

3. **Ans. A:** Secretion of ACTH is mainly under nervous control and corticotrophin releasing hormone control (CRH). Trauma via reticular formation, emotions via limbic system, diurnal variation from suprachiasmatic nucleus increase CRH secretion. (AK Jain 731)

4. **Ans. B:** Increase in aldosterone or Conn's syndrome levels leads to rise Na+ levels and fall in K+. The patient has muscular weakness, hypokalemic nephropathy and metabolic alkalosis that may precipitate tetany. These are features of Addison's disease. (AK Jain 743)

5. **Ans. B:** Calcitonin exerts its calcium lowering activity by inhibiting osteoclastic activity, i.e., bone resorption and decreases renal formation of 1,25 DHCC. (AK Jain 719)

6. **Ans. C:** Myxoedema is characterized by swelling of skin and subcutaneous tissue, goiter, i.e., enlargement of thyroid gland, puffiness of face with periorbital swelling, coarseness and loss of scalp hair, dry thickened yellow skin, low ESR. (AK Jain 701)

7. **Ans. D:** Hyperthyroidism is characterized by exopthalmos (protrusion of eyeballs), lid retraction, increase in BMR (upto 100%), heat intolerance, tachycardia. (AK Jain 702, 703)

8. **Ans. C:** Parathyroid glands are essential for life, as their removal can cause death from asphyxia, resulting in spasm of laryngeal muscles, thoracic muscles and diaphragm. PTH increases plasma Ca++ and decreases plasma phosphate by promoting bone resorption. It increases action of cAMP in bone and kidney. (AK Jain 716)

9. **Ans. C:** Cushing's syndrome has centripetal deposition of fat (extremities are thin) – fat metabolism, diabetes mellitus (hyperglycemia), poor wound healing, polycythemia, increase platelet count, eosinopenia. (AK Jain 738)

10. **Ans. D:** Progesterone is a C_{21} steroid. The major source is corpus luteum and placenta and minor source is testes and adrenal cortex. (AK Jain 824)

11. **Ans. A:** Epinephrine is three times more potent than NE to produce hyperglycemia as β adrenergic action predominates. Epinephrine increases glycogenolysis in the liver, skeletal muscle and adipose tissue. The increased glucose is used in fight, flight and fright reactions, as described by Canon. (AK Jain 755)

12. **Ans. B:** Circulating oestrogens are conjugated in the liver to form water soluble sulphates and glucoronides which are then excreted. 65% are excreted in the urine, 80% which is excreted as *oestrone* and *oestriol*; and 20% remaining as oestradiol. 10% excreted in faeces. The fate of remaining 25% is not known. (AK Jain 822)
13. **Ans. C:** FSH is secreted by Gonadotrophs along with LH. Gonadotrophs are Basophils, that stain blue or green with basic dyes. They account for 20% of chromophils (granular secretory cells of anterior pituitary). (AK Jain 667)
14. **Ans. D:** Sertoli cells are glycogen rich nourishing cells that secrete androgen binding protein, inhibin, MRF. They also secrete an enzyme aromatase that converts androgens to oestrogen. They control release of mature spems into lumen of seminiferous tubules. They also provide for the blood testes barrier. (AK Jain 793, 807, 808, 810, 816)
15. **Ans. B:** Antidiuretic hormone facilitates water absorption via V_2 receptors in collecting ducts; concentrating urine. Its absence leads to deficient faculatative absorption of water. (AK Jain 681)
16. **Ans. A:** Loss of negative feedback from T_3 and T_4 leads to increase TSH on thyroidectomy. TSH increases on exposure to cold, prolonged anxiety, prolonged excitement. TSH decreases during warmth, stress, anxiety and excitement. (AK Jain 694)
17. **Ans. A:** Increased HCO_3 reabsorption causes metabolic alkalosis called *hypokalemic alkalosis*, this decreases free ionized Ca++ which may precipitate tetany. (AK Jain 741)
18. **Ans. B:** Factors that increase GH are substrate deficiency, e.g., Hypoglycemia, Oestrogen, Increased amino acid levels (infusion of arginine), Glucagon, stress, deprivation of REM sleep, Dopamine and its agonists. GH inhibition occurs by GH itself, Glucocorticoids, Glucose, REM sleep, FFA. (AK Jain 668)
19. **Ans. B:** Patient with chromaffin secreting tumors of adrenal medulla (phaeo-cromocytoma) secretes both epinephrine and norepinephrine. They have high level of BP (300/200 mm Hg), increase BMR, headache, sweating, palpitation. If alpha blocker like phentolamine is given it results in dramatic fall in blood pressure. This test is also used to diagnose phaechrocmocytoma. (AK Jain 757)
20. **Ans. D:** Decrease in aldosterone levels leads to Na+ excretion and K+ retention. The patient has hypotension , pigmentation of skin, unable to withstand stress. These are features of Addison's disease. (AK Jain 744)
21. **Ans. A:** Smooth endoplasmic reticulum or Agranular ER is the site of synthesis of steroid in adrenal cortex and the site of detoxifying processes in other cells. The sarcoplasmic reticulum plays an important role in skeletal muscle and cardiac muscles. (AK Jain 7)
22. **Ans. D:** Insulin increases glucose entry into tissues of skeletal muscles, cardiac muscle and smooth muscle, adipose tissues, WBC, liver, mammary glands, alpha cell of pancreatic of islet. (AK Jain 767)
23. **Ans. B:** SIADH or Syndrome of Inappropriate ADH secretion is characterized by water retention, increased blood volume, decreased aldosterone secretion, hypernaturia and hyponatremia, decreased urinary excretion of water, increased urine osmolality, shift of water in ICF, water intoxication or overhydration. (AK Jain 681)

24. **Ans. A:** Prolactin inhibiting factor is Dopamine in nature. It is more important than PRH. Prolactin is regulated by PIH and PRH from hypothalamus. (AK Jain 679)

25. **Ans. B:** Increase in number of receptors or affinity occurs in starvation and exercise. This enables glucose to enter the cells with little or no insulin. (AK Jain 769)

26. **Ans. B:** Vasomotor changes are common like flushing of skin of face, neck and upper chest called Hot flashes, i.e., sensation of warmth. They coincide with LH surge. (AK Jain 825)

27. **Ans. B:** Estrogen lowers plasma cholesterol (increase HDL), preventing development of atherosclerosis, promoting growth of internal and external genitalia. (AK Jain 823)

28. **Ans. B:** Steroid hormones and thyroid hormones being lipid soluble can easily enter target cells and exert their effect by combining to a specific *cytoplasmic* receptor protein. Hormone receptor complex bind to DNA at HRE or hormone responsive element promoting synthesis of enzymes. Most proteins and polypeptide homones cannot cross the lipid cell membrane and bind to cell membrane receptor. They activate adenyl cyclase increasing cAMP in the cells. (AK Jain 661)

29. **Ans. A:** Insulin is a large polypeptide containing 51 amino acids, containing two chains. It is secreted from beta cells at rate of 1-2 U/hour. It causes synthesis of glycogen by activating glycogen synthetase. Insulin stimulates lipoprotein lipase and deposition of triglycerides in muscles, adipose tissue and liver. (AK Jain 762,768,769)

30. **Ans. D:** Testosterone produces protein anabolic and growth promoting effect by (a) increases synthesis and deposition of protein in skeletal muscles (b) increases libido and has a role in growth spurt (c) causes epiphyses to fuse, stopping linear growth. (AK Jain 814)

31. **Ans. C:** Prolactin inhibiting factor ceases to act on transaction of pituitary stalk, as a result prolactin increases. Other characteristic features of pituitary insufficiency include features secondary to GH, thyroid and adrenal insufficiency, gonadal hypoplasia and myxoedema. (AK Jain 685)

32. **Ans. A:** Choline + acetyl CoA are combined in the presynaptic membrane to form acetylcholine that is stored in clear vesicles. (AK Jain 159)

33. **Ans. A:** NE containing neurons in the brain are located in the locus cerulus and brainstem. NE acts as inhibitory neurotransmitters in the thalamus, cerebral and cerebellar cortex, as a mood elevator, secretion of anterior pituitary hormones, regulation of ADH, oxytocin and control of body temperature. (AK Jain 1079)

34. **Ans. B:** Effects of sympathetic ANS system are produced by adrenergic receptor for, e.g., alpha 1 receptor contracts radial muscle of iris to produce dilatation. (AK Jain 72)

35. **Ans. A:** GHIH or somatostatin decrease GH secretion. GHIH is released from hypothalamus, nerve endings in brain, cells of antrum of stomach, and delta cells of pancreatic islets of Langerhans. It also blocks the synthesis of insulin, glucagons and gastrin, producing a state of hypoglycemia. Hypothalamic gonadotophin releasing hormone (GnRH) help release FSH, LH (Gonadotrophins) from anterior pituitary. (AK Jain 669, 803)

36. **Ans. A:** Endocrine glands liberate their secretions into the blood stream to be

carried to act on distant organs and tissues. Also, living tissues contain many substances which may be activated in certain circumstances to exert profound effects in immediate neighborhood. Such substances which act at the sites of their synthesis and release have been called *Local Hormones.* Examples include: Acetylcholine, Histamine, 5-hydroxytryptamine (serotonin), prostaglandins, adenosine derivatives: AMP, ADP and ATP, Plasma polypeptides, e.g., angiotensin, plasma kinins. (AK Jain 781-785)

37. **Ans. B:** Acetylcholine is rapidly removed from its site of action by diffusion and acetylcholinesterase. It is a local hormone that acts in heart muscle, cilia of heart muscle. (AK Jain 781, 1076)

38. **Ans. A:** Adenohypophysis or Anterior pituitary consists of pars distalis (anterior pituitary), pars tuberalis (pituitary stalk), pars intermedia (intermediate lobe). Adenohypophysis is influenced by hormones which come from the hypothalamus via portal vessels (hypothalamo hypophyseal portal vessels). The hormones are FSH, ACTH, LH, TSH and GH from Anterior pituitary. Intermediate lobe secrete melanocyte stimulating hormone. Posterior lobe or Neurohypophysis secrete vasopressin (ADH) and Oxytocin. (AK Jain 665, 666)

39. **Ans. C:** Thyroid cells synthesize glycoprotein thyroglobulin, which is stored as colloid in the follicles. T3 and T4 are bound to TBG by peptide linkages and stored. (AK Jain 687, 690, 692)

40. **Ans. D:** Insulin lack causes Hyperglycemia, when renal threshold exceeds 180 mg%, glyocosuria occurs, due to osmotic diuresis, Polyuria occurs, water and sodium loss causes dehydration and increased thirst, polydipsia. Increased glucagon secretion causes hyperglycemia by stimulating glycogenolysis and gluconeogenesis. It is a catabolic hormone, a hormone of energy release. (AK Jain 761, 773)

41. **Ans. D:** Hyperthyoidism features include tachycardia, high output cardiac failure, exertional dyspnea due to excessive beta adrenergic stimulation. Thyrotoxic myopathy, weight loss, creatinuria and negative nitrogen balance due to protein catabolism secondary to increase in BMR, hypercalciuria or calcium loss in urine due to mobilization of bone protein leading to osteoporosis. (AK Jain 696, 705)

42. **Ans. B:** Thyroxine causes increased heat production or calorigenic action secondary to stimulation of oxygen consumption, increasing BMR. Thyroxine decreases serum cholesterol (normal 150-240 mg%) by increasing breakdown of cholesterol in the liver and by increasing excretion of cholesterol in bile. Thyroxine potentiates the action of epinephrine and norepinephrine and their action on CNS and CVS can be decreased by sympathectomy or injection of β blocking agents. (AK Jain 696, 699)

43. **Ans. B:** Menopause is the period of life when menstruation naturally ceases. The ovaries become smaller, the graffian follicles disappear. The changes are due to senile changes in the ovary which no longer reacts to the stimulatory effect of hormones (especially gonadotrophins). Therefore, the ovaries no longer secrete 17 β oestradiol. The pituitary gonadotrophins actually increase. (AK Jain 825)

44. **Ans. B:** Aldosterone secretion is regulated by hyponatremia, hyperkalemia, circadian rhythm, ANP (Extra Renal Control Mechanism) and Intra Renal Mechanism, e.g., sympathetic nervous system,

hypovolemia, acute hypotension, chronic disorders associated with oedema, e.g., cirrhosis of liver. (AK Jain 741)

45. **Ans. A:** Phytates in diet decreases calcium reabsorption. Excess of inorganic phosphate, oxalate or phytic acid-convert Ca++ into insoluble unabsorbable form. High protein, acidity in the stomach increases calcium absorption from GIT. Normal serum calcium is 9-11 mg%. Normal calcium occurs in two forms: Diffusable: 55%, (a) Ionized Ca++ or free Ca++ in body fluids (4.72 mg%). It is physiologically active. Its level chiefly depends on Ca++ reabsorption from GIT. 1,25 DHCC increases serum calcium and phosphate by its action on GIT, bones and kidney. On GIT it acts on nuclei of intestinal epithelial cells to increase calbindin D that binds Calcium to increase its absorption. (AK Jain 709, 710, 715)

46. **Ans. D:** Role of ACTH in secretion of aldosterone is minimal. Injection of large doses of ACTH increases aldosterone secretion which falls in 1-2 days even with increasing dose of ACTH injection. This is because of decrease in renin secretion secondarily to fall in ECF volume. Aldosterone secretion is regulated by hyponatremia, hyperkalemia, circadian rhythm, ANP (Extra Renal Control Mechanism) and Intra Renal Mechanism, e.g., sympathetic nervous system, hypvolemia, acute hypotension, chronic disorders associated with oedema, e.g., cirrhosis of liver. (AK Jain 741)

47. **Ans. D:** Renin Angiotensin causes increase aldosterone secretion from zona glomerulosa of adrenal cortex. That causes decrease in renal sodium excretion, and increase in blood volume. Increased arteriolar tone results from action of angiotensin on blood vessels. (AK Jain 742)

48. **Ans. B:** Calcium metabolism is mainly dependent on Parathormone. PTH gives the human being a new skeleton by bone remodeling in ten years. The main effects of PTH are hypercalcaemia and hypophosphataemia. GH and thyroid hormone have a minor role in increasing calcium. Calcitonin protects against postprandial hypercalemia and has a minor role in protecting the bones of the mother during pregnancy. (AK Jain 717, 719)

49. **Ans. B:** Cerebral blood flow is autoregulated between blood pressures 65 to 140 mm Hg mean BP. This is chiefly dependennt on PO_2 and PCO_2 values. It is steady in the recumbent position, upright position, coughing and straining at stools. (AK Jain 364) Evidently epinephrine has a little role to play. (AK Jain 364)

50. **Ans. C:** NE acts mainly on α receptors, and on β1 receptors. It has no action on β2 receptors. The mechanism on α 1 receptors is via release of intracellular calcium. The mechanism of action on α 2 receptors is reduction in cAMP concentrations. G proteins or GTP (Guanosine Tri phosphate) are membrane bound regulatory proteins having three subunits: α, β and γ. The α subunit modulates the activity by interacting with adenyl cyclase, interacting with phospholipase C, directly opening an ion channel. (AK Jain 17, 953)

51. **Ans. C:** Steroid hormones and thyroid hormones being lipid soluble can easily enter target cells and exert their effect by combining to a specific *cytoplasmic* receptor protein. Hormone receptor complex bind to DNA at HRE or hormone responsive element promoting synthesis of enzymes. Most proteins and polypeptide homones cannot cross the lipid cell membrane and bind to cell membrane

receptor. They activate adenyl cyclase increasing cAMP in the cells. (AK Jain 661)

52. **Ans. B:** Cerebral blood flow is auto-regulated between blood pressures 65 to 140 mm Hg mean BP. This is chiefly dependent on PO_2 and PCO_2 values. It is steady in the recumbent position, upright position, coughing and straining at stools. (AK Jain 364). Evidently epinephrine has a little role to play. (AK Jain 364)

53. **Ans. A:** Insulin is a polypeptide of 51 amino acids. A chain contains 21 amino acids and B chain 30 amino acids. The insulin from cattle or sheep is liable to evoke formation of antibodies in man which cause allergic reactions whereas pig insulin, which is more closely linked is better tolerated. (AK Jain 762)

54. **Ans. A:** Testosterone major action is spermatogenesis. It is responsible for development of secondary sexual organs. It produces increase in protein anabolism and growth promoting effect by causing nitrogen retention in body, calcium sulphate retention. Testosterone stimulates erythropoietin to cause increase erythropoiesis not haemopoiesis. (AK Jain 814, 815)

55. **Ans. C:** Other Circadian rhythms include melatonin secretion, ACTH and Glucocorticoid secretion and bronchial tone. (AK Jain 426, 731, 780, 1036)

56. **Ans. C:** Once diabetic ketoacidosis occurs there is marked resistance to insulin, due to presence of large amounts of FFA, which decreases utilization of glucose. (AK Jain 772-773)

57. **Ans. D:** Prolactin inhibiting factor is Dopamine in nature. It is more important than PRH. It is regulated by PIH and PRH from hypothalamus. Prolactin inhibiting factor ceases to act on transaction of pituitary stalk, as a result prolactin increases. Thus D is the best choice. (AK Jain 679)

58. **Ans. A:** Gluconeogenesis is the formation of glucose or glycogen from non carbohydrate sources. Glucagon promotes formation of glucose from lactate, pyruvate, glycerol and amino acids producing slower but more sustained rise in blood sugar. (AK Jain 761)

59. **Ans. D:** The sensitivity of the uterus to oxytocin increases during latter part of pregnancy and is greatest just before the onset of labour. The concentration of plasma oestrogen increases and that of progesterone decreases during last few weeks of pregnancy. During the first stage of labour the amniotic fluid contains PGE1 and PGE2a. (AK Jain 849)

60. **Ans. B:** Testosterone is secreted from cholesterol in the Leydig cells of testis. Seminiferous tubules are sites of spermatogenesis. (AK Jain 814)

61. **Ans. B:** Steroid hormones and thyroid hormones being lipid soluble can easily enter target cells and exert their effect by combining to a specific *cytoplasmic* receptor protein. Hormone receptor complex bind to DNA at HRE or hormone responsive element promoting synthesis of enzymes. Most proteins and polypeptide homones cannot cross the lipid cell membrane and bind to cell membrane receptor. They activate adenyl cyclase increasing cAMP in the cells. (AK Jain 661)

62. **Ans. C:** If the stimulus is subthreshold, action potential is not produced and muscle does not contract. (AK Jain 34)

63. **Ans. D:** Somatostatin does not inhibit prolactin. Prolactin inhibiting factor is Dopamine in nature. It is more important than PRH. It is regulated by PIH and PRH from hypothalamus. (AK Jain 679)

64. **Ans. A:** Experimental diabetes is caused by Alloxan by destroying beta cells to decrease insulin secretion. (AK Jain 766)

65. **Ans. C:** 5 Hydroxy tryptamine or serotonin is formed from tryptophan. It gives rise to melatonin or N-acetyl-5-methoxytryptamine in pineal gland. (AK Jain 779)

66. **Ans. B:** Hormonal control of insulin secretion: Thyroid hormone, glucocorticoids, oral contraceptives (oestrogen and progesterone preparations), *in pharmacological doses* increases blood glucose, which by producing β cell exhaustion decrease insulin secretion and also depress glucose induced insulin secretion. GH directly stimulates β cell to increase insulin secretion. Epinephrine acts directly on beta cells of the pancreas, which have more α receptors, and decreases cAMP and thus insulin secretion decreases. (AK Jain 765)

67. **Ans. A:** Aldosterone secretion is regulated by angiotensin, hyponatremia, hyperkalemia, circadian rhythm, ANP (Extra Renal Control Mechanism) and Intra Renal Mechanism, e.g., sympathetic nervous system, hypovolemia, acute hypotension, chronic disorders associated with oedema, e.g., cirrhosis of liver. (AK Jain 741)

68. **Ans. C:** The layers of the adrenal cortex are memorized by the pneumonic GFR from outside to inside, i.e., Glomerulosa, Fasciculata, Reticularis. They secrete from inside to outside AGM (assistant general manager), i.e., Adrenal steroids (androgens), Glucocorticoids (cortisol) and Mineralocorticoids (aldosterone). The adrenal medulla secretes norepinephrine. (AK Jain 725)

69. **Ans. B:** As in 68.

70. **Ans. A:** As in 68.

71. **Ans. D:** As in 68.

72. **Ans. D:** The hormones are FSH, ACTH, LH, TSH and GH from Anterior pituitary. Intermediate lobe secrete melanocyte stimulating hormone. Posterior lobe or Neurohypophysis secretes vasopressin (ADH) and Oxytocin. (AK Jain 665, 666)

73. **Ans. A:** 17 β estradiol is the most potent. Most of the C_{19} steroids which have got a keto- group at 17 positions are called 17 ketosteroids. (AK Jain 727)

74. **Ans. A:** The hormones are FSH, ACTH, LH (ICSH), TSH and GH from Anterior pituitary. Intermediate lobe secrete melanocyte stimulating hormone. Posterior lobe or Neurohypophysis secrete vasopressin (ADH) and Oxytocin. (AK Jain 665, 666)

75. **Ans. C:** Metyrapone test is for pituitary ACTH reserve estimation. Drug metyraone inhibits 11 β hydroxylase in the adrenal cortex and thereby interferes with the synthesis of cortisol. This decreases cortisol, increases ACTH which increases sex hormone synthesis normally. (AK Jain 746)

76. **Ans. B:** Testosterone is synthesized from cholesterol that gives rise to Pregnenolone, that gives rise to aldosterone, cortisone and oestradiol. (AK Jain 728)

77. **Ans. A:** Luteinizing hormone (LH) or interstitial cell stimulating hormone (ICSH) stimulates ovulation and luteinization of ovarian follicles in female and testosterone secretion in male. (AK Jain 803)

78. **Ans. B:** Steroid hormones and thyroid hormones being lipid soluble can easily enter target cells and exert their effect by combining to a specific *cytoplasmic* receptor protein. Hormone receptor complex bind to DNA at HRE or hormone responsive element promoting synthesis of enzymes. Most proteins and polypeptide homones cannot cross the lipid cell

membrane and bind to cell membrane receptor. They activate adenyl cyclase increasing cAMP in the cells. (AK Jain 661)

79. **Ans. B:** Substance P is a transmitter for afferent neurons that relay sensory information into the CNS and is thought to be involved in the transmission of nociceptive (pain producing) stimuli. It is found in high concentrations in the endings of primary afferent neurons (Aδ and C fibers) in the spinal cord, in nigrostriatal system, in the hypothalamus. (AK Jain 1082)

80. **Ans. B:** Also, living tissues contain many substances which may be activated in certain circumstances to exert profound effects in immediate neighborhood. Such substances which act at the sites of their synthesis and release have been called *Local Hormones*. Examples include: Acetylcholine, Histamine, 5-hydroxytryptamine (serotonin), prostaglandins, adenosine derivatives: AMP, ADP and ATP, Plasma polypeptides, e.g., angiotensin, plasma kinins. Most of these play a role in the small intestine, e.g., 5HT secreted from argentaffin cells. (AK Jain 781-785)

81. **Ans. D:** Gastrinoma are gastrin producing tumors which can occur in stomach or duodenum or pancreatic tumour of δ cells (Zollinger-Ellison syndrome). These tumors secrete large amounts of gastrin which causes excessive secretion of HCl that predisposes to peptic ulcer. Gastrin is secreted by G cells or gastrin cells from deeper portions of pyloric glands. It occurs in 3 forms. (AK Jain 221)

82. **Ans. D:** Haemorrhage decreases blood volume and discharge from atrio-caval receptors and this increases ADH secretion. Renal ischemia decreases GFR and increases rennin angiotensin system from JG apparatus. Decrease in tissue perfusion increases aldosterone secretion from adrenal cortex. (AK Jain 412)

83. **Ans. A:** Aldosterone secretion is regulated by hyponatremia, hyperkalemia, circadian rhythm, ANP (Extra Renal Control, Mechanism) and Intra Renal Mechanism e.g., sympathetic nervous system, hypovolemia, acute hypotension, chronic disorders associated with oedema, e.g., cirrhosis of liver. (AK Jain 741)

84. **Ans. C:** Decrease in aldosterone levels leads to Na+ excretion and K+ retention. The patient has hypotension and fall in blood volume. (AK Jain 744)

85. **Ans. B:** Removal of adrenal glands leads to sodium and water loss due to loss of aldosterone, decreasing ECF and produces hypotension, dehydration, circulatoy collapse and death. (AK Jain 739)

86. **Ans. D:** Contraction of pyloric sphincter occurs via sympathetic nerves supplying it. It is a local response and acts via α1 receptor. (AK Jain 955)

87. **Ans. A:** Hypersecretion of catecholamines is seen in tumors of chromaffin tissue. These tumors contain benign and large amounts of Epinephrine and Norepineprine. The features include sustained or paroxysmal hypertension, BP rises upto 300/200 mm Hg. (AK Jain 757)

88. **Ans. D:** Alpha or A cells secrete Glucagon, beta or B cells secrete insulin. Delta or D cells secrete Somatostatin (GHIH) and in small amounts Gastrin. F cells secrete pancreatic polypeptide. (AK Jain 760)

89. **Ans. B:** Carbonic anhydrase helps form bicarbonic acid. Carbonic anhydrase inhibitors are acetoxolamide, decrease H_2CO_3 formation, decreasing H+ secretion, increasing K+ secretion and decreasing bicarbonate reabsoption. (AK Jain 543)

90. **Ans. C:** Type II cells *(granular pneumocytes)* are thicker and contain numerous lamellar inclusion bodies which secrete surfactant. The maturation of surfactant occurs is accelerated by glucocorticoids. Near term the cortisol levels in both fetus and mother goes up. The number of receptors for cortisol in the lung also increases. (AK Jain 426, 440)

91. **Ans. D:** Testosterone major action is spermatogenesis. It is responsible for development of secondary sexual organs. It produces increase in protein anabolism and growth promoting effect by causing nitrogen retention in body, calcium sulphate retention. Testosterone stimulates erythropoietin to cause increase erythropoiesis and not haemopoiesis. Ejaculation is a neural phenomenon involving internal pudendal nerve as afferent and hypogastric nerve as efferent. (AK Jain 814, 815)

92. **Ans. B:** Vitamin D_3 is cholecalciferol. In the body it is converted to a more important physiologically active hormone 1,25 dihydroxycholecalciferol (1,25 DHCC). (AK Jain 715)

93. **Ans. B:** The main effects of PTH are hypercalcemia and hypophosphataemia. It also increases bone resorption, increases number of osteoclasts and osteoblasts on bone surface. (AK Jain 717)

94. **Ans. A:** Steroid hormones and thyroid hormones being lipid soluble can easily enter target cells and exert their effect by combining to a specific *cytoplasmic* receptor protein. Hormone receptor complex bind to DNA at HRE or hormone responsive element promoting synthesis of enzymes. Most proteins and polypeptide hormones cannot cross the lipid cell membrane and bind to cell membrane receptor. They activate adenyl cyclase increasing cAMP in the cells. (AK Jain 661)

95. **Ans. A:** Growth hormone, glucocorticoids, glucose, REM sleep, FFA decrease the secretion of growth hormone. Substrate deficiency, oestrogen, increased amino acids, glucagons, stress, deprivation of REM sleep, dopamine increase growth hormone secretion. (AK Jain 668)

96. **Ans. C:** Glucocorticoids have anti-inflammatory and antiallergic actions. They prevent tissue damage by stabilizing lysosomal membrane, thereby preventing escape of protease and hydrolase enzymes into the tissue fluid. This blocs the systemic effects of bacterial toxins by preventing damage to neighboring tissues. (AK Jain 737)

97. **Ans. A:** TSH acts via thyroid receptors increasing cAMP. The effects of TSH is to increase I^- trapping mechanism, increases organic binding of I^- to tyrosine, increases number and size of thyroid cells, increases proteolysis of thyroglobulin, i.e., increases released of stored T_4, T_3 and increases blood flow to the thyroid gland. (AK Jain 693)

98. **Ans. D:** T_3 and T_4 are iodine containing amino acids , tyrosine are stored in thyroid follicle bound to thyroglobulin. Calcitonin is secreted by parafollicular cells or "C cells" which lie between follicular cells. (AK Jain 688)

99. **Ans. D:** Endothelial cells form three similar polypeptides endothelins I, II and III. The Endothelin 1 (ET-1) being the most potent vasoconstrictor agent which acts via ET_A receptors. It produces vasoconstriction in many body tissues. (AK Jain 336)

100. **Ans. B:** Hyperthyoidism features include tachycardia, high output cardiac failure, exertional dyspnea due to excessive

beta adrenergic stimulation. Thyrotoxic myopathy, weight loss, creatinuria and negative nitrogen balance due to protein catabolism secondary to increase in BMR, hypercalciuria or calcium loss in urine due to mobilization of bone protein leading to osteoporosis. (AK Jain 696, 705)

101. **Ans. D:** Prolactin inhibiting factor ceases to act on transaction of pituitary stalk or blockage of hypothalamic-hypophyseal venous portal system, as a result prolactin increases. Other characteristic features of pituitary insufficiency include features secondary to GH, thyroid and adrenal insufficiency, gonadal hypoplasia and myxoedema. (AK Jain 685)

102. **Ans. B:** Menopause is the period of life when menstruation naturally ceases. The ovaries become smaller, the graffian follicles disappear. The changes are due to senile changes in the ovary which no longer reacts to the stimulatory effect of hormones (especially gonadotrophins). Therefore, the ovaries no longer secrete 17 β oestradiol. The pituitary gonadotrophins FSH, LH actually increase. (AK Jain 825)

103. **Ans. A:** Increased arteriolar tone results from action of angiotensin on blood vessels. (AK Jain 742)

104. **Ans. A:** Receptors for endorphins are sites of action of opiate drugs morphine and codeine. They are present in substantia gelatinosa that conveys information of pain. There are of three types beta-endorphins, dynorphins and enkephalins. Beta endorphins act by increasing K+ permeability hyperpolarizing neurons in CNS and primary afferents. (AK Jain 929,1081)

105. **Ans. B:** Tyrosine forms dopamine that forms norepinephrine which gives rise to Epinephrine in the adrenal medulla. 5 Hydroxy tryptamine or serotonin is formed from tryptophan. It gives rise to melatonin or N-acetyl-5-methoxytryptamine. (AK Jain 749,779)

106. **Ans. A:** The foetus and the placenta interact as a functional unit, called fetoplacental unit in the formation of oestrogen and progesterone. Oestriol, the predominant oestrogen of pregnancy, originates from the fetal adrenal cortex, which forms DHEA. Therefore, the urinary oestriol excretion of the mother can be monitored as an index of the state of the fetus development. (AK Jain 845)

107. **Ans. A:** Progesterone is a thermogenic hormone. Recording the basal body temperature before passing urine in the morning is an index of time of ovulation. In the pre-ovulatory phase the oral BBT is 36.3 to 36.8 °C which increases by 0.3-0.5 °C after ovulation. (AK Jain 826)

108. **Ans. A:** Decrease in aldosterone levels leads to Na+ excretion and K+ retention. The patient has hypotension and fall in blood volume. (AK Jain 744)

109. **Ans. A:** Thyroid follicles is made up of multiple acini or follicles, 50-500 µm in diameter. Thyroid cells synthesize thyroid hormones by iodide trapping, coupling and storage. (AK Jain 687)

110. **Ans. A:** Calcitonin is secreted by parafollicular cells or "C cells" which lie between follicular cells. Calcitonin exerts its calcium lowering activity by inhibiting osteoclastic activity, i.e., bone resorption and decreases renal formation of 1,25 DHCC. (AK Jain 688, 719)

111. **Ans. A:** Pituitary is called the master gland of the body. Anterior pituitary secrete hormones FSH, ACTH, LH, TSH and GH (FALTS pneumonic). Intermediate lobe secrete melanocyte stimulating hormone. Posterior lobe or Neurohypophysis secrete vasopressin (ADH) and Oxytocin. (AK Jain 665, 666)

112. **Ans. B:** Na+ and Cl- is extruded out of thick ascending limb helps operate the counter current multiplier. In excretion of dilute urine requires normal function of the loop of Henle (especially the tic acending limb), distal tubule, adequate delivery of fluid to these regions, absence of ADH, reduced medullary interstitium. (Ganong 721)

113. **Ans. A:** Emotions lie anger, anxiety, apprehension, fear, fatigue, frustration act via limbic system (amygdaloid nucleus) to reach hypothalamus and increases ACTH secretion from anterior pituitary to increase glucocorticoid secretion. Aldosterone secretion is regulated by Intra Renal Mechanism, e.g., sympathetic nervous system, e.g., anxiety. (AK Jain 733, 741)

114. **Ans. A:** Calcitonin is secreted by parafollicular cells or "C cells" which lie between follicular cells of thyroid gland. (AK Jain 688)

115. **Ans. D:** Hypoglycemia occurs when blood glucose falls less than 60 mg%. The causes are due to insulin overdose, or overdose of oral hypoglycemic agents, beta islet cell adenoma or hyperplasia, severe exercise in diabetic mellitus patients. (AK Jain 774)

116. **Ans. C:** During each cycle, of approx. a month's time, some 10-15 follicles enlarge to become secondary follicles under the influence of FSH from the anterior pituitary. (AK Jain 826-829)

117. **Ans. C:** Blood brain barrier applies to the barrier between blood and the brain tissue. The endothelial cells are surrounded by a continuous belt of tight junctions that do not permit substances of more than molecular weight of 2000 to pass. Glucose is the major source of energy for neurons. It is transported across the walls of brain capillaries via glucose transporter–GLUT 1. (AK Jain 394-395)

118. **Ans. B:** Vitamin D acts on GIT: intestinal epithelial cells nuclei to increase synthesis of calbindin D that binds calcium to increase its absorption. (AK Jain 715)

119. **Ans. B:** Glucose transport across the following cells does not require insulin:
   (a) Brain except ventromedial nucleus of hypothalamus.
   (b) Kidney tubules, GIT and RBC's.

   Thus brain cannot withstand hypoglycemia. In diabetic patients glucose absorption from Kidney tubules, GIT and RBC's remain unaffected. (AK Jain 767)

120. **Ans. D:** Calcitonin exerts its calcium lowering activity by inhibiting osteoclastic activity, i.e., bone resorption and decreases renal formation of 1,25 DHCC. Calcitonin protects against postprandial hypercalcemia and has a minor role in protecting the bones of the mother during pregnancy. (AK Jain 719)

121. **Ans. A:** Testosterone is secreted from cholesterol in the Leydig cells of testis. Seminiferous tubules are sites of spermatogenesis. (AK Jain 814)

122. **Ans. C:** Cerebral oxygen consumption is 3.3 ml/100 gm/min or 45 ml/min, i.e., 20% of whole body at rest. This is fairly constant and is not affected by thyroxine. Cerebral blood flow is regulated at arterial pressure of 65 and 140 mm Hg. Noradrenergic discharge helps to regulate pressure between 65-200 mm Hg (plateau phase is extended to right). Vasodilator hydralazine and ACE inhibitor captopril reduce the length of the plateau. (Ganong 610)

123. **Ans. A:** Oestriol, the predominant oestrogen of pregnancy, originates from the fetal adrenal cortex, which forms DHEA. Therefore, the urinary oestriol

excretion of the mother can be monitored as an index of the state of the fetus development. (AK Jain 845)

124. **Ans. C:** Glucocorticoid prevents peripheral utilization of glucose by inhibiting phosphorylation and exerting anti-insulin action on peripheral tissues. This increases blood glucose. (AK Jain 734)

125. **Ans. A:** Luteinizing hormone (LH) or interstitial cell stimulating hormone (ICSH) stimulates ovulation and luteinization of ovarian follicles in female and testosterone secretion in male. (AK Jain 803)

126. **Ans. C:** Glucocorticoid produces lymphopenia due to decrease in lymphocyte mitotic activity by interfering with DNA synthesis and increased lymphocyte destruction in the circulation (directly), thus increased uric acid excretion in the urine. (AK Jain 735)

127. **Ans. D:** The patient has hypotension, pigmentation of skin, unable to withstand stress. These are features of Addison's disease. (AK Jain 744)

128. **Ans. A:** One of the mechanisms by which chemical messengers in ECF bring changes in cell function are by activating phospholipase C that forms Inositol phosphate (IP_3) which diffuses to the endoplasmic reticulum, where it triggers the release of Calcium into the cell to produce physiological effects. (AK Jain 20, 21)

129. **Ans. B: Parathyroid hormone (PTH):** Arguably the most crucial hormone for magnesium homeostasis, PTH directly increases magnesium reabsorption in the kidneys, influencing overall levels. Low PTH can lead to increased magnesium excretion. **Calcitonin:** This hormone, primarily involved in calcium regulation, also promotes magnesium reabsorption in the kidneys and synergizes with PTH in certain situations. **Antidiuretic hormone (ADH):** ADH indirectly modulates magnesium reabsorption by influencing water reabsorption in the kidneys. Higher ADH creates a concentration gradient that enhances magnesium reabsorption alongside water.

Brenner and Rector's The Kidney, 11th Edition (Chapter 14: Disorders of Magnesium Homeostasis) Primer on Kidney Diseases, 8th Edition (Chapter 10: Disorders of Magnesium Metabolism).

130. **Ans. D:** Theca interna cells of graffian follicles secrete oestrogens. These cells have many LH receptors. The other sources are placenta, adrenal cortex, testis and placenta. (AK Jain 822)

131. **Ans. C:** FSH is secreted by Gonadotrophs of anterior pituitary along with LH. (AK Jain 667)

132. **Ans. A:** Thyroxine causes increased heat production or calorigenic action secondary to stimulation of oxygen consumption, increasing BMR. Thyroxine levels are index of metabolic state. (AK Jain 696, 699)

133. **Ans. C:** FSH controls spermatogenesis by its direct stimulating action on the seminiferous tubules. It is necessary for the maintenance of an optimal level of spermatogenic activity. At any given moment some areas of seminiferous epithelium are active while others are at rest. (AK Jain 810, 815)

134. **Ans. A:** Prolactin inhibiting factor is Dopamine in nature. It is more important than PRH. It is regulated by PIH and PRH from hypothalamus. (AK Jain 679)

135. **Ans. D:** Insulin causes synthesis of glycogen by activating glycogen

synthetase. Insulin stimulates lipoprotein lipase and deposition of triglycerides in muscles, adipose tissue and liver and glycolysis for utilization of glucose in peripheral cells. (AK Jain 762,768,769)

136. **Ans. C:** Reverse T3 is 3,3[1] ,5[1]T3. It is an inactive form of triiodo thyronine or 3,5,3[1] T3, formed by the oxidative condensation of DIT +MIT. (AK Jain 690)

137. **Ans. D:** Most proteins and polypeptide hormones cannot cross the lipid cell membrane and bind to cell membrane receptor. They activate adenyl cyclase increasing cAMP in the cells. However, epinephrine acts directly on beta cells of the pancreas, which have more *α receptors*, and decreases cAMP and thus insulin secretion decreases. (AK Jain 661, 765)

138. **Ans. D:** Progesterone is a thermogenic hormone that is secreted in the luteal phase that lasts for a fixed period of fourteen days. Recording the basal body temperature before passing urine in the morning is an index of time of ovulation. In the pre-ovulatory phase the oral BBT is 36.3 to 36.8°C which increases by 0.3-0.5°C after ovulation. (AK Jain 826)

139. **Ans. A:** Role of ACTH in secretion of aldosterone is minimal. Injection of large doses of ACTH increases aldosterone secretion which falls in 1-2 days even with increasing dose of ACTH injection. This is because of decrease in rennin secretion secondarily to fall in ECF volume. ACTH acts to help convert cholesterol acetate to pregnenolone. ACTH helps to increase synthesis of glucocorticoids in Zona fasciculata. (AK Jain 741)

140. **Ans. B:** ADH is a hypothalamic hormone synthesized in the cells of the supraoptic nucleus which are called magnocelluar neurosecretory neuron in response to hyperosmolarity. (AK Jain 679, 680)

141. **Ans. C:** Cushing's syndrome or hypercortisolism shows features of centripetal distribution of fat, poor wound healing (protein metabolism), moon facies, buffalo hump, purple striae. (AK Jain 737, 738)

142. **Ans. C:** Thyroxine has a negative feedback mechanism to decrease TSH secretion from pituitary. (AK Jain 694)

143. **Ans. B:** ACTH secretion is minimum between 6 and 9 p.m. in the evening and is maximum between 6 and 9 a.m. in the morning. (AK Jain 732)

144. **Ans. A:** Characteristic features of pituitary insufficiency include features secondary to GH, thyroid and adrenal insufficiency, gonadal hypoplasia and myxoedema and increased sensitivity to insulin. (AK Jain 685)

145. **Ans. A:** Oestrogen prevents osteoporosis by inhibiting effects of cytokines (IL-1 and IL-6) on osteoclasts. In postmenopausal women decreased oestrogen concentration leads to increased sensitivity of bone to PTH. Osteoporosis is a condition which leads to decrease in all constituents of bone, which leads to decrease in bone mass with preservation of normal ratio of mineral to matrix. It occurs due to a relative excess of osteoclastic function. (AK Jain 714)

146. **Ans. B:** Insulin secretion is increased by glucose that gets metabolized in the islet cells. (AK Jain 767)

147. **Ans. C:** FSH is secreted by Gonadotrophs along with LH. Gonadotrophs are Basophils, that stain blue or green with basic dyes. They account for 20% of chromophils (granular secretory cells of anterior pituitary). (AK Jain 667)

148. **Ans. C:** Thyroxine causes increased heat production or calorigenic action

secondary to stimulation of oxygen consumption, increasing BMR. Thyroxine decreases serum cholesterol (normal 150-240 mg %) by increasing breakdown of cholesterol in the liver and by increasing excretion of cholesterol in bile. Thyroxine potentiates the action of epinephrine and norepinephrine and their action on CNS and CVS can be decreased by sympathectomy or injection of β blocking agents. (AK Jain 696, 699)

149. **Ans. D:** Steroid hormones and thyroid hormones being lipid soluble can easily enter target cells and exert their effect by combining to a specific *cytoplasmic* receptor protein. Hormone receptor complex bind to DNA at HRE or hormone responsive element promoting synthesis of enzymes. Most proteins and polypeptide homones cannot cross the lipid cell membrane and bind to cell membrane receptor. They activate adenyl cyclase increasing cAMP in the cells. (AK Jain 661)

150. **Ans. B:** Progesterone promotes the growth of lobules and alveolar tissue in the breasts. It decreases the excitability of myometrial cells, it inhibits ovulation by inhibiting release of GnRH from hypothalamus. Progesterone is a thermogenic hormone. Recording the basal body temperature before passing urine in the morning is an index of time of ovulation. In the pre-ovulatory phase the oral BBT is 36.3 to 36.8°C which increases by 0.3-0.5°C after ovulation. (AK Jain 824, 826, 864)

151. **Ans. D:** 20-day is luteal phase. Progesterone is a thermogenic hormone that is secreted in the luteal phase that lasts for a fixed period of fourteen days. After ovulation as the corpus luteum forms, serum progesterone concentration increases. LH and FSH levels fall. (AK Jain 826, 829, 830)

152. **Ans. A:** Under the influence of ADH only 10-12% of filtered water is reabsorbed. 75-80% of water reabsorption occurs in the PCT across osmotic gradient set by active transport of solutes. (AK Jain 545)

153. **Ans. A:** Thyroxine causes increased heat production or calorigenic action secondary to stimulation of oxygen consumption, increasing BMR. Thyroxine decreases in myxoedema, patient has cold intolerance. (AK Jain 696, 699)

CHAPTER 5

Kidney

What is Important in Kidney?

Kidney Function Tests, Structure and Physiology of a Nephron

1. **Active reabsorption of glucose occurs in:**
   A. Proximal tubule
   B. Loop of Henle
   C. Distal tubule
   D. All of the above

2. **GFR is:**
   A. Plasma filtered through microtubules
   B. Serum filtered through microtubules
   C. Arterial blood filtered through microtubules
   D. Venous blood filtered through microtubules

3. **The acute control response to increased extracellular fluid volume involves or is associated with all of the following except:**
   A. Increased urine osmolarity
   B. Stretch of the two atria
   C. Decreased sympathetic stimulations of kidneys
   D. Decreased secretion of antidiuretic hormone

4. **All of the following are actively reabsorbed from the proximal tubules except:**
   A. Sodium
   B. Urea
   C. Amino acids
   D. Urea and water

Following test results were obtained from a person over a 24-hour period:

I. Urine flow rate:1.0 ml/min
II. Urine inulin:100 mg/100 ml
III. Plasma inulin:1.0 mg/100 ml
IV. Urine urea: 200 mmol/L
V. Plasma urea: 5 mmol/L

5. **What is the urea clearance?**
   A. 4.4 ml/min B. 88 ml/min
   C. 440 ml/min D. 44 ml/min

6. **What is glomerular filtration rate?**
   A. 100 ml/min B. 125 ml/min
   C. 150 ml/min D. 175 ml/min

7. **Glomerular filtration rate can be increased by:**

A. Increased arterial blood pressure
B. Increased the plasma protein concentration
C. Efferent arteriolar dilation
D. Afferent arteriolar constriction

8. **Tubular membrane is maximum permeable to:**
A. Creatinine B. Inulin
C. Urea D. Sucrose

9. **Normal kidney does not allow passage of:**
A. β-globuli B. Inulin
C. Urea D. Sucrose

10. **GFR is increased when:**
A. Plasma oncotic pressure is increased
B. Glomerular hydrostatic pressure is decreased
C. Tubular hydrostatic pressure is increased
D. Increased renal blood flow

11. **Which of the following has no T_m value?**
A. Albumin, arginine
B. Beta hydroxybutyrate, glucose
C. Glucose haemoglobin, phosphate
D. Urea

12. **Which substance is actively transported by the tubular cells but has not been shown to have a Tm?**
A. Albumin
B. Haemoglobin
C. Both albumin and haemoglobin
D. Sodium ions

13. **Which of the following is minimally excreted in urine?**
A. Urea B. Creatinine
C. Uric acid D. Chloride

14. **Where in the kidney, does active reabsorption of sodium ions occur?**
A. Collecting duct
B. Distal tubule
C. Ascending limb of Henle
D. Only B and C

15. **In a normal adult the desire for micturition is felt when and how much urine fills the bladder?**
A. 100-200 cc B. 300-400 cc
C. 600-800 cc D. 1000 cc

16. **Two substances that can probably be used to determine filtration fraction are:**
A. Inulin and mannitol
B. Urea and diodrast
C. PAH and phenol red
D. Inulin and PAH

17. **Normal urinary protein excretion is:**
A. 50-150 mg% B. 150-250 mg%
C. 250-500 mg% D. Nil

18. **Which of the following is truly physiological?**
A. Mild pedal edema
B. Increased GFR
C. Albuminuria
D. Increased BP

19. **Inulin clearance closely resembles:**
A. GFR
B. Renal plasma flow
C. Creatinine clearance
D. PAH clearance

20. **Juxtamedullary nephrons in kidney are what percentage of total nephrons?**
A. 15 B. 50
C. 70 D. 90

21. **Water is not freely permeable but sodium and potassium are in which portion of nephron?**
    A. Thick ascending limb
    B. Descending limb
    C. DCT
    D. Collecting tubules

22. **Which is true regarding Renin secretion?**
    A. Increase K+ in PCT, Increase in Renin
    B. Decrease in Na+ in DCT, Increase in Renin secretion
    C. Inversely proportional to the potassium levels
    D. Directly proportional to the ADH levels

23. **True is:**
    A. Creatine has the lowest clearance measure GFR most accurately
    B. Creatine clearance is 70 ml/min
    C. Creatinine is a sensitive endogenous index of renal function
    D. Creatine has no relation to blood urea

24. **Potassium is:**
    A. Entirely absorbed in the PCT
    B. Completes with Na+ absorption
    C. Absorption depends upon aldosterone
    D. Mainly absorbed in the DCT

25. **Which of the following has the lowest clearance in human kidney?**
    A. Creatinine B. K+
    C. Cl- D. Glucose

26. **Addis test is used for:**
    A. Urinary sodium
    B. Urinary sediment
    C. Blood lactate
    D. Serum Magnesium

27. **Normal creatinine clearance (in L/24 hours):**
    A. 46-76 B. 76-116
    C. 116-148 D. 148-168

28. **Sodium movement in PCT from lumen to tubular cells:**
    A. Active process
    B. Passive process
    C. Filtration
    D. Associated with H_2O

29. **The hyperosmolarity of the renal medulla is due to increased content of:**
    A. K+ B. Na+ and urea
    C. Glucose D. Na+

30. **Total area of glomerular capillary endothelium across which filtration occurs in humans is:**
    A. 0.1 sq m B. 0.4 sq m
    C. 0.8 sq m D. 1.2 sq m

31. **Urine/Plasma ratio of Na^+ (meq/L) is:**
    A. 0 B. 1
    C. 10 D. 100

32. **Urine/Plasma ratio of glucose in mg/dl is:**
    A. 0 B. 1
    C. 10 D. 100

33. **In humans, % of the nephrons having long loops:**
    A. 5 B. 15
    C. 35 D. 65

34. **The length of distal convoluted tubule is .... mm.**
    A. 2 B. 5
    C. 8 D. 12

35. **Total length of nephrons including the collecting ducts ranges from ....mm.**

A. 5-10 B. 25-45
C. 45-65 D. 65-100

36. **The volume of blood in the renal capillaries at any given time is:**

A. 30-40 ml B. 70-100 ml
C. 100-300 ml D. 300-450 ml

37. **Renal blood flow is (L/min):**

A. 0.8-1.2 B. 1.2-1.3
C. 1.5-2.0 D. 2.0-2.5

38. **In humans, effective renal blood flow is:**

A. 425 B. 525
C. 625 D. 725

39. **A-V O_2 difference in kidney is .... ml/l of blood.**

A. 14 B. 18
C. 62 D. 114

40. **Oxygen consumption of human kidney is about ...... ml/min.**

A. 9 B. 12
C. 18 D. 62

41. **Creatinine is not ideal to measure GFR in humans because:**

A. It is toxic
B. It is secreted by tubules and some may be reabsorbed
C. Not freely filtered
D. Affects filtration rate

42. **Oxygen consumption of renal cortex and inner medulla are....... ml/100g/min respectively.**

A. 9,4 B. 4,9
C. 9,0.4 D. 0.4,6

43. **Which of the following is not true about inulin?**

A. A polymer of fructose
B. Molecular weight 5200
C. Found in dahlia tubers
D. None of the above

44. **The following are the characteristics of substance suitable for measuring GFR except:**

A. Freely filtered
B. Stored in kidney
C. Not reabsorbed or excreted by tubules
D. Not protein bound

45. **The following is the minor factor affecting GFR:**

A. Partial nephrectomy
B. Ureteric obstruction
C. Diabetes insipidus
D. Hypoproteinemia

46. **Factors affecting GFR are:**

A. Changes in renal blood flow
B. Changes in glomerular capillary hydrostatic pressure
C. Ureteric obstruction
D. All of the above

47. **Sodium filtered per minute (microequivalents) is:**

A. 21825 B. 18125
C. 18060 D. 14585

48. **Ethyl alcohol produces diuresis by:**

A. Producing osmotic diuresis
B. Inhibiting vasopressin secretion
C. Decreases tubular absorption of Na^+
D. Inhibits Cl- absorption

49. **When GFR falls, the sodium excretion will:**

A. Increase
B. Fall
C. Fall followed by increased
D. No change

50. The following inhibits Cl- reabsorption in the loop of Henle except:

A. Thiazide B. Furosemide
C. Ethacrynic acid D. Triamterene

51. Which one of the following is not responsible for concentration of urine in the kidney:

A. Aldosterone B. Angiotensin II
C. Vasopressin D. Epinephrine

52. Renin secretion is increased by following except:

A. Hypovolemia
B. Hyponatremia in PCT
C. Hyponatremia in DCT
D. Sympathetic stimulation

53. In DCT, following are absorbed by following are absorbed except:

A. Na^+ B. K^+
C. Water D. Cl-

54. Glucose is transported through:

A. Na antiport
B. Na cotransport
C. K antiport
D. K symport

55. Maximal urine acidity is:

A. 0.0003 B. 0.003
C. 0.03 D. 3.0

56. The daily loss of nitrogen in urine is approximately:

A. 2-5 B. 5-10
C. 10-20 D. 25-50

57. All of the following factors stimulate the release of Renin following trauma except:

A. Vasopressin release
B. Decreased renal perfusion pressure
C. Fall in circulating blood volume
D. Increased sympathetic stimulation of adrenals

58. Following is least absorbable in tubules:

A. Creatinine B. Glucose
C. Urea D. Sucrose

59. Which of the following changes would not occur, under steady-state conditions in a normal person as a result of a 50% decrease in sodium intake?

A. Increased plasma concentration of angiotensin II
B. Increased plasma Aldosterone concentration
C. Approximately a 50% decrease in sodium excretion
D. A large (greater than 10%) decrease in plasma sodium concentration

60. A substance which has a renal clearance 20 times that of inulin is probably:

A. Only filtered at glomeruli
B. Only secreted by tubules
C. Filtered and reabsorbed
D. Synthesized in tubules and secreted

61. Site of action of ADH is:

A. Glomerulus of nephron
B. Proximal convoluted tubule
C. Distal convoluted tubule
D. Collecting duct

62. **Each kidney contains about...... nephrons.**

A. One million B. Two million
C. Four million D. ½ million

63. **In renal glycosuria, the renal threshold for glucose is:**

A. Low
B. High
C. Same
D. Greatly increased

64. **Active reabsorption of glucose appears to occur in:**

A. Distal tubule
B. Loop of Henle
C. Proximal tubule
D. All of the above

65. **A substance commonly used to measure renal blood flow is:**

A. Glucose
B. Cobalt labeled red cells
C. Inulin
D. Para-aminohippuric acid

66. **Which of the following pressure changes leads to an increased GFR:**

A. Increase arterial plasma colloid osmotic pressure
B. Increase glomerular capillary hydrostatic pressure
C. Increase hydrostatic pressure in Bowman's capsule
D. Increase net filtration pressure

67. **One of the following does not form filtration barrier in nephron:**

A. Mesangium
B. Specialised endothelium
C. Endothelial cell
D. Basement membrane

68. **Urine plasma ratio of creatinine (mg/dl) is:**

A. 0 B. 1
C. 60 D. 150

69. **Relaxation of Mesangial cells of kidney is brought about by:**

A. cAMP
B. Endothelin
C. PGF2
D. Vasopressin

70. **Following cells are responsible for acid secretion in kidney:**

A. T cells B. P cells
C. Mesangial cells D. Pericytes

71. **Renin activity in elderly:**

A. High B. Low
C. No change D. A or B

72. **Max absorption of glucose in elderly:**

A. 370 B. 150
C. 180 D. 120

73. **The sodium content of the filtrate in renal medulla is very high because:**

A. At the loop of Henle, there is counter current mechanisms
B. Increased blood flow to vasa recta
C. Increased absorption of sodium from PCT
D. Increased excretion of Na from PCT

74. **Which is true about rennin:**

A. It helps to convert angiotensinogen to Angiotensin1
B. Secreted by PCT
C. Increase GFR increase secretion of rennin
D. Decrease Plasma and Water

75. **Amino acids are completely absorbed in:**
A. PCT B. DCT
C. CT D. All of the above

76. **Acidification of urine takes place in:**
A. PCT
B. DCT
C. Collecting duct
D. Asc. Loop of Henle

77. **Diluting segment of a nephron is:**
A. Thin ascending limb of loop of Henle
B. Thick ascending limb of loop of Henle
C. Medullary collecting duct

78. **The renal threshold value for complete tubular reabsorption of glucose is:**
A. 70-80 mg% blood glucose
B. 120-140 mg%
C. 170-180 mg%
D. 220-240 mg%

79. **In the nephron, reabsorption of most of the filtered water occurs in the:**
A. Proximal convoluted tubule
B. Loop of Henle
C. Distal convoluted tubule
D. Collecting duct

80. **Counter current mechanism of the kidney consists of:**
A. Proximal tubule and collecting tubule
B. Loop of Henle and vasa recta
C. Collecting tubule and vasa recta
D. Proximal tubule and loop of Henle

81. **Match List I (Tubular function) with List II (Substance) and select the correct answer:**

List I	List II
A. Active reabsorption	1. Urea
B. Passive diffusion	2. Phenol red
C. Secretion	3. Glucose
D. Neither reabsorption nor secretion	4. Inulin

	A	B	C	D
A.	3	1	4	2
B.	1	3	2	4
C.	3	1	2	4
D.	1	3	2	4

82. **True statement regarding oxygen consumption in the kidney is:**
A. Oxygen consumption decreases as blood flow decreases
B. Oxygen consumption in maximum in renal medulla
C. Oxygen consumption in ml/min is maximum as compared to any organ in the body
D. Consumption is equal in both cortex and medulla

83. **Sertoli cells secrete following except:**
A. Mullerian inhibiting substance
B. Somatomedin
C. Inhibin
D. Androgen binding protein

84. **Loop of Henle absorbs the following except:**
A. Na^+ B. K^+
C. Cl^- D. Urea

85. **The diuretic group that does not require access to the tubular lumen to induce diuresis is:**
A. Carbonic anhydrase inhibitor

B. Na-Cl symport inhibitor

C. Mineralocorticoid antagonist

D. Na-K symport inhibitor

86. The Renal plasma (RPF) of a patient was to be estimated through the measurement of para-aminohippuric acid (PAH) clearance. The technician observed the procedures correctly but due to an error in the weighing inadvertently used thrice the recommended dose of PAH. The RPF estimated is likely to be:

A. False-high

B. False-low

C. False high or false low depending on the GFR

D. Correct and is unaffected by PAH overdose

87. Normal urine flow and voiding pressure is:

A. 15 ml/min and < 60 mm Hg

B. 10-15 ml/min and 60-80 mm Hg

C. <10 ml/min and >60 mm Hg

D. 15 ml/min and > 60 mm Hg

88. All the following are true about uric acid excretion except:

A. It is filtered at the glomerulus

B. It is completely reabsorbed in PCT

C. It is resecreted in the loop of Henle

D. Effectively 50% of the filtered uric acid is excreted

EXPLANATORY ANSWERS OF KIDNEY

1. **Ans. A:** Glucose, amino acids and bicarbonate are reabsorbed with Na+ in the early portion of the proximal tubule. (Ganong 713)
2. **Ans. A:** GFR is approximately 125 ml/min. (Ganong 709)
3. **Ans. A:** Sympathetic stimulation decreases urine output. ADH decreases urine output. ANP increases urine output (Naturesis). (Ganong 733, 734).
4. **Ans. D:** Urea contributes to establishment of the osmotic gradient in medullary pyramids and to the ability forming a concentrated urine in collecting duct. (Ganong 721)
5. **Ans. D:** $C_{urea} = (U_{urea} \times V)/P_{urea} = (200 \times 1)/5 = 40$ ml/mn. (Ganong 709)
6. **Ans. B:** GFR is approximately 125 ml/min or 7.5 l/h or 180 l/d. (Ganong 709)
7. **Ans. A:** GFR= $K_f(P_{GC} - P_T) - (\pi_{GC} - \pi_T)$. K_f is the glomerular ultracoefficient, P_{GC} is the hydrostatic pressure in the glomerular capillaries, P_T the hydrostatic pressure in tubule, π_{GC} and π_T the osmotic pressure in the glomerular capillaries and tubule, respectively. (Ganong 709)
8. **Ans. B:** Inulin, a polymer of fructose with a molecular weight of 5,200 is found in dahlia tubers. It is freely filtered, neither reabsorbed nor secreted in the tubules. (Ganong 709)
9. **Ans. B:** The amount of protein in the urine is <100/d that comes from the tubular cells. (Ganong 709)
10. **Ans. D:** GFR=$K_f(P_{GC} - P_T) - (\pi_{GC} - \pi_T)$. K_f is the glomerular ultracoefficient, P_{GC} is the hydrostatic pressure in the glomerular capillaries, P_T the hydrostatic pressure in tubule, π_{GC} and π_T the osmotic pressure in the glomerular capillaries and tubule, respectively. (Ganong 709)
11. **Ans. D:** Renal active transport systems have a maximal rate or transport maximum (Tm) at which they can transport a particular substance. Urea transport is mediated by urea transporters, primarily by facilitated diffusion, and not actively. Thus Tm value is zero. (Ganong 712)
12. **Ans. D:** Na+ is actively transported out of all parts of the renal tubule except the thin portions of the loop of Henle by various transport proteins. The Tm value for Na systems is high and it is difficult to saturate them. (Ganong 713)
13. **Ans. C:** Urine concentrations are as follows: Uric acid 5 mmol/d, Urea 410 mmol/d, Creatinine 12 mmol/d, Cl- 150 mg/d. (Ganong 713)
14. **Ans. D:** In the collecting duct is a Na+ channel (ENaC) that uptakes Na. In the distal tubule NaCl cotransporters exists and in the TAL Na+, 2 Cl-, K+ cotransporter along with Na+/H+ exchanger. (Ganong 714)
15. **Ans. B:** The first urge to void is felt at volume of 150 ml and a marked sense of fullness at about 400 ml. (Ganong 731)
16. **Ans. D:** Inulin is used to measure GFR and PAH renal plasma flow. Filtration fraction = GFR/PAH and is normally 0.16-0.20. (Ganong 711)
17. **Ans. A:** Normal amount of protein in the urine is less than 100 mg/d and most is not filtered but comes from tubular cells. (Ganong 710)
18. **Ans. B:** GFR changes linearly with changes in renal blood flow (directly propotional). (Ganong 710)

19. **Ans. A:** Inulin is freely filtered and neither absorbed nor secreted in the tubules. (Ganong 709)
20. **Ans. D:** Juxtamedullary nephrons have longer loops and thin ascending limbs. They are involved in countercurrent mechanism and concentrate urine. (Ganong 721)
21. **Ans. A:** The thin descending limb is permeable to water but not to NaCl. The thin ascending limb is relatively impermeable to water but permeable to Na+ and Cl-. (Ganong 721)
22. **Ans. B:** Renin secretion is increased by decrease in Na + in DCT, decrease afferent arteriolar pressure, Angiotensin II, and Vasopressin. It is stimulated by increased sympathetic activity, increased circulating catecholamines, prostaglandins. (Ganong 462)
23. **Ans. C:** Clearance of creatinine can be used to determine GFR, as only some creatinine is secreted by tubules, and is a worthwhile index of renal function. (Ganong 709)
24. **Ans. A:** Potassium is removed from the tubular fluid by active reabsorption in the proximal tubules (Table 38.5). (Ganong 713, 727)
25. **Ans. D:** Clearance is defined as the volume of substance that is cleared of the substance by the kidney. Glucose clearance is less than inulin which is less than creatinine which is less than PAH. (Ganong 709)
26. **Ans. B:** Urinary sediment containing hyaline casts shows destruction of glomeruli or tubular cells. Presence of granular casts, RBC, bacteria, glucose, albumin and ketone bodies is abnormal. (AK Jain 580)
27. **Ans. C:** Creatine clearance is 80-110 ml/min. Determination of 24-hour endogenous creatinine clearance is an approximate estimate of GFR (180L/d). (AK Jain 548)
28. **Ans. A:** Sodium is actively transported out of all parts of the renal tubule except thin portions of loop of Henle. (Ganong 713)
29. **Ans. B:** Urea contributes to the establishment of the osmotic gradient in the medullary pyramids and to the ability to form a concentrated urine in collecting ducts. Na+ and Cl- out of thick ascending limb helps operate the counter current multiplier. (Ganong 721)
30. **Ans. C:** Glomerular capillary forms 3-6 capillary loops in six lobules, i.e., 20-40 loops in all. Endothelium of glomerular capillaries is fenestrated with pores of 100 nm in diameter. (Ganong 726)
31. **Ans. A:** Normally 96% to well over 99% of filtered Na+ is reabsorbed. (Ganong 726)
32. **Ans. A:** Urine contains no glucose normally. Glucose appears in urine when concentration exceeds 180 mg/dl. (Ganong 714)
33. **Ans. B:** 15% of humans have juxtamedullary nephrons in long loops that extend down in the medullary pyramids. (Ganong 703)
34. **Ans. B:** Length in mm of: PCT=15, Loop of Henle =14-26, DCT=5, CD=20. (AK Jain 515)
35. **Ans. C:** They are approximately 1 to 1.3 million nephrons in each kidney. Total length of nephron ranges from 45 to 65 mm. (AK Jain 515)
36. **Ans. A:** Total surface area of renal capillaries is equal to the total surface area of the tubules=12 m^2. The volume of blood in the renal capillaries at any given time is 30-40 ml. (AK Jain 524)
37. **Ans. B:** Under basal conditions renal blood flow is (300-400 ml/100 g min) or 1.2 to 1. L/min. It is very high as compared to flow through other body organs. (AK Jain 525)

38. **Ans. C:** ERPF=$(U_{PAH}V)/P_{PAH}$ is measured by clearance of PAH and averages 625 ml/min. (Ganong 707)
39. **Ans. A:** (A-V) O_2 difference in kidney is 1.5 ml% is low. Venous blood has high pO_2 and is 80-85% saturated with oxygen. (AK Jain 525)
40. **Ans. C:** O_2 consumption of kidney is about 18-20 ml/min or (6 ml/100 gm/min) which represents 8% of VO_2 of whole body at rest. (AK Jain 525)
41. **Ans. B:** In primates, including humans, some creatine is secreted by tubules and some may be reabsorbed. In addition, plasma creatinine levels are inaccurate at low creatinine levels because the method for determining creatinine measures small amounts of other plasma constituents. But it is used as a worthwhile index of renal function. (Ganong 709)
42. **Ans. C:** O_2 consumption of kidney is about 18-20 ml/min or 6 ml/100 g/min. The cortex has 9 ml/100 g/min and inner medulla 0.4 ml/100 gm/min is due to oxygen consumption (VO_2). High cortical blood flow is due to the fact that it contains major components of nephron. (AK Jain 525-526)
43. **Ans. D:** Inulin is a polymer of fructose with a molecular weight of 5200 found in dahlia tubers used to measure GFR. (Ganong 709)
44. **Ans. B:** It is freely filtered, neither reabsorbed nor secreted in the tubules, a substance suitable for measuring GFR, should be non toxic and not metabolized by body. (Ganong 709)
45. **Ans. B:** Ureteric obstruction increases the hydrostatic pressure in Bowman's capsule, along with edema of kidney inside tight renal capsule. (Table 38.4, Ganong 711)
46. **Ans. D:** Factors affecting GFR are changes in renal blood flow, changes in glomerular capillary hydrostatic pressure, changes in hydrostatic pressure in Bowman's capsule, changes in concentration of plasma protein, changes in Kf. (Table 38.4, Ganong 711)
47. **Ans. B:** Sodium filtered per minute is 26,000/ per 24 hours or 18125 microequivalents per minute. (Ganong 713)
48. **Ans. B:** Ethanol inhibits vasopressin secretion that explain diuretic action after alcohol. (Ganong 728)
49. **Ans. D:** When GFR flow increases , increase in reabsorption of solutes in proximal tubule so that percentage of tubule solute absorbed is held constant. (Glomerulotubular balance). (Ganong 715-716)
50. **Ans. D:** Triamterene (pyrenium) is a potassium sparing diuretic and inhibit the action of spironolactone, inhibiting Na+/ K+ exchange in Collecting duct. Loop diuretics such as furosemide (Lasix), ethacrynic acid (Edicein) and bumeanide inhibits the Na+ K+ 2 Cl- cotransporter in the medullary thick ascending limbs of loop of Henle. Metolazone, thiazines such as Chlorothiazine (Diuril) inhibit Na+Cl- cotransporters in the early portion of distal tubules. (Ganong 728, Table 38.11)
51. **Ans. D:** Angiotensin II, Aldosterone causes Na+ reabsorption. Vasopressin causes water Reabsorption. (AK Jain 679)
52. **Ans. B:** Renin secretion is decreased by increased Na+ and Cl- reabsorption across macula densa. Increased afferent arteriolar pressure, Angiotensin II and Vasopressin. (Ganong 462, Table 24.1)
53. **Ans. B:** Much of the filtered K+ is removed from tubular fluid by active reabsorption in proximal tubules and K+ is then secreted into the fluid by distal tubular cells. (Ganong 727)
54. **Ans. B:** Glucose, amino acids and bicarbonate are reabsorbed along with Na+ (cotransport) in the early portion of the proximal tubule. (Ganong 713)

55. **Ans. C:** Urine pH ranges from 4.5 to 8.0 (average 6-6.5), slight acidic, therefore turns blue litmus red. After meals it may become alkaline. (AK Jain 724, Ganong 579)

56. **Ans. D:** Urea is 20-30 g/d, Uric Acid 0.6 g/d, Creatinine 1.2 g/d. (AK Jain 520)

57. **Ans. D:** Renin secretion is decreased by increased Na+ and Cl- reabsorption across macula densa. Increased afferent arteriolar pressure, Angiotensin II and Vasopressin (Ganong 462, Table 24.1). Renin secretion is increased by sympathetic activity via renal nerves, increased circulating catecholamines, prostaglandins. (Ganong 462)

58. **Ans. A:** Creatinine is least absorbable in kidneys. Glucose is actively absorbed and Urea passively reabsorbed. (AK Jain 508)

59. **Ans. D:** Angiotensin and Aldosterone is stimulated by hyponatremia. They restore Na back to normal concentration by decreasing excretion. (AK Jain 538)

60. **Ans. D:** Clearance is defined as the volume of substance that is cleared of the substance by the kidney. Inulin is only filtered. A substance that is cleared 20 times faster than inulin would be both synthesized and secreted by the tubules. Clearance = Filtered + Secreted. (AK Jain 548)

61. **Ans. D:** Site of action of ADH is collecting duct. Higher the plasma ADH level, greater would be the concentration of urine formed and less its volume. Results in the excretion of low volume, hypertonic urine. Absence of ADH, results in dilute tubular fluid entering the DCT and collecting tubule. It remains hypotonic and is excreted as high volume, hypotonic urine. (A K Jain 556)

62. **Ans. A:** Each kidney has one million nephrons, which are the functional unit. (AK Jain 515)

63. **Ans. A:** In renal glycosuria the renal threshold for glucose is low, that is why glucose appears more in urine. The actual renal threshold is 200 mg% of arterial plasma and 180 mg% of venous plasma (Because 20 mg% gets utilized while passing through the tissues). (AK Jain 536)

64. **Ans. C:** Glucose, amino acids and bicarbonate are reabsorbed along with Na+ (cotransport) in the early portion of the proximal tubule. (Ganong 713)

65. **Ans. D:** ERPF $=(U_{PAH}V)/P_{PAH}$ is measured by clearance of PAH and averages 625 ml/min. (Ganong 707)

66. **Ans. B:** Due to constriction of efferent arteriole, Renal plasma flow reduces, that increases hydrostatic pressure, that leads to increase in GFR. (AK Jain 533)

67. **Ans. A:** The two layers separating blood from the glomerular filtrate in Bowman's capsule: The capillary endothelium and specialized epithelium. These are separated by basal lamina. Stellate cells are located between the basal lamina and endothelium. The glomerular membrane is made of five layers:

Layer 1: Foot processes of podocytes.

Layer 2: Lamina rara externa or outer cement layer.

Layer 3: Lamina densa forms the basement membrane.

Layer 4: Lamina rara interna.

Layer 5: Endothelial cell layer is fenestrated with pores of 100 nm in diameter.

These features allow plasma filtration with retention of plasma proteins and blood cells. (AK Jain 516, 517)

68. **Ans. D:** Urine plasma ratio of creatinine is 150.

69. **Ans. A:** Relaxation of Mesangial cells of kidney is brought about by ANP (Atrial natriuretic peptide), cAMP, Dopamine, PGE_2. These increase GFR. Endothelins, PGF_2 (prostaglandins), ADH (Vasopressin), Histamine, Leukotriens C and D, Norepinephrine, Platelet activating factor, Platelet-derived growth factor, Thromboxane A_2 causes contraction of mesangial cells and decreases GFR. (AK Jain 532, 568)

70. **Ans. A:** Following cells are responsible for acid secretion in the kidney (T cells) mainly in DCT and Collecting tubule. (AK Jain 562)

71. **Ans. A:** Renin activity in elderly is high. Renin helps regulate BP (i.e., increases). For elderly BP is high, so rennin activity also increases. (AK Jain 523)

72. **Ans. A:** Transport Maximum (Tm): Renal transport refers maximal amount of a given solute that can be transported (reabsorbed or secreted) per minute by renal tubules. Tm for glucose is approximately 75 mg/min in male and 300 mg/min in female. (AK Jain 712)

73. **Ans. A:** The sodium content of the filtrate in renal medulla is very high. This is due to the counter current multiplier operating at the loop of Henle. The descending limb of Henle is impermeable to solute. The ascending limb of Henle is impermeable to water. By activity of Na+2 K+ Cl- cotransporter some solute enters the medullary interstitium. Also urea absorbed from collecting duct helps make the medulla hyperosmolar. (AK Jain 555)

74. **Ans. A:** Renin helps in conversion of Angiotensinogen to Angiotensin I. (AK Jain 522)

75. **Ans. A:** Amino acids are completely reabsorbed into the proximal convoluted tubule. (A K Jain 530)

76. **Ans. B:** Acidification of urine occurs in DCT and Collecting tubule. (AK Jain 562)

77. **Ans. B:** The thick ascending limb is relatively impermeable to water but permeable to Na+ and Cl-. The urine becomes hypotonic here. (Ganong 721)

78. **Ans. C:** The actual renal threshold is 200 mg% of arterial plasma and 180 mg% of venous plasma (Because 20 mg % gets utilized while passing though the tissues). (AK Jain 536)

79. **Ans. A:** Glucose, amino acids and bicarbonate are reabsorbed along with Na+ (cotransport) in the early portion of the proximal tubule. (Ganong 713)

80. **Ans. B:** Na+ and Cl- is extruded out of thick ascending limb helps operate the counter current multiplier. Urea contributes to the establishment of the osmotic gradient in the medullary pyramids and to the ability to form a concentrated urine in collecting ducts. The vasa recta forms the countercurrent exchanger, maintaining this gradient. (Ganong 721)

81. **Ans. C:** Glucose is actively reabsorbed, Urea passively diffuses from collecting duct to add to the medullary hyperosmolarity, Phenol red is secreted and inulin neither reabsorbed nor secreted. Inulin is thus used to measure GFR. (AK Jain 510, 520, 529)

82. **Ans. A:** Oxygen extraction or A-V difference does not change in kidney despite massive alterations indicating Oxygen consumption varies directly with blood flow. Oxygen consumption of kidney (V_{O2}) is about 18-20 ml/min (6 ml/100 gm/min) which represents 8% of V_{O2} of whole body at rest (normal: 250 ml/min), second to the heart (8-10 ml/100 gm/min). Blood flow and V_{O2}max within the kidneys is not homogenous because cortical flow is more than that of medulla. High cortical flow is because cortex contains major part of the nephrons. Low blood flow of the medulla is because of the

high resistance of vasa recta and increase viscosity of blood at the hair pin bend. (AK Jain 498)

83. **Ans. B:** Sertoli cells are large complex glycogen containing cells that stretch from the basal lamina to the lumen. The spermatids mature into spermatozoa in deep folds of the cytoplasm of the Sertoli cells. The sertoli cells secrete Androgen-binding protein (ABP), inhibin and MIS. They do not synthesize androgens, but contain aromatase (CYP19), enzyme responsible for conversion of androgens to estrogen. ABP functions to maintain a high stable supply of androgen in the tubular fluid. Inhibin inhibits FSH secretion, causes regression of the mullerian ducts in males during fetal life. (Ganong 428, 430)

84. **Ans. B:** The loop of Henle consists of a descending limb which arises in continuity with the terminal part of the PCT. Descending limb continues into the thin segment where the epithelium is of attenuated flat cells. From the thin segment arises the thick ascending limb. Loop of Henle actively transports Na+ and Cl- out of its thic ascending limb. The thin descending limb transports water. Urea transport is mediated by four urea transporters. (AK Jain 519, 555)

85. **Ans. C:** Carbonic anhydrase inhibitor, e.g., acetozolamide (Diamox) decreases carbonic anhydrase activity, decreasing intracellular H_2CO_3 formation, decreasing H^+ formation within tubular cells. There other actions are to decrease H+ secretion, increase K+ secretion and decreasing HCO_3^- reabsorption.

Inhibition of Na+ Cl- cotransport in DCT, e.g., Thiazides (Diuril, Esidrex). Hypokalemia is a major side effect.

Na-K-2Cl- cotransport (symport) in the thick ascending limb of loop of Henle, e.g., Furosemide (Lasix), Ethacrynic acid (Edecrin), Bumetanide (Bumet) are popularly called loop Diuretics. Hypokalemia is a major side effect.

Inhibition of Na+-K+ exchange in collecting ducts by inhibiting aldosterone or Na channels (ENa C), e.g., Spironolactone (Midamox, Bidiret) is the most commonly used diuretic in clinical practice. It is a K+ sparing diuretic. They do not produce hypokalemia. (AK Jain 560)

86. **Ans. D:** When PAH is infused at low doses 90% of the PAH is removed in a single Circulation through the kidney. (Ganong 707)

87. **Ans. A:** Normal voiding pressure is 20 cm of H_2O, normal volume 1-2.5 l/d average 1.5 l/d. (AK Jain 578)

88. **Ans. A:** 50 mmol/d is filtered, 49 mmol/d is reabsorbed in proximal tubule, 4 mmol/d is Secreted, i.e., 98% is reabsorbed. (Ganong 713)

CHAPTER 6

Blood

What is Important in Blood?

Production and Function of Important Blood Components, Haemostasis and Blood Coagulation

1. **In polycythemia, the increase in blood pressure is due to increase in:**
   A. Blood volume
   B. Peripheral resistance
   C. Thyroxine
   D. Renin

2. **Vitamin K is required for the synthesis of factors:**
   A. VII
   B. IX
   C. X
   D. All of the above

3. **Carbonic anhydrase in RBC forms:**
   A. Oxyhemoglobin
   B. Carboxyhemoglobin
   C. HCO_3^- in blood
   D. Carbaminohemoglobin

4. **When osmotic fragility is normal, RBC's begin to hemolyse when suspended in saline:**
   A. 0.33% B. 0.48%
   C. 0.9% D. 1.2%

5. **Endothelial cells synthesize:**
   A. Fibrinogen B. Factor VIII
   C. Factor X D. Factor XII

6. **Adult hemoglobin has chains:**
   A. 2α, 2γ B. 2α, 2β
   C. 4α D. 2α

7. **Iron is stored in:**
   A. RBC
   B. Reticuloendothelial system
   C. Plasma
   D. All of the above

8. **For cyanosis to be manifested, the amount of reduced hemoglobin in blood, should be:**
   A. 1 gm% B. 3 gm%
   C. 5 gm% D. 7 gm%

9. **Freezing point of normal human plasma is:**
   A. 4°C B. 0°C
   C. -0.54°C D. -1.54°C

10. **In which of the following, bleeding time is characteristically increased:**

A. Von Willebrand's disease
B. Hemophilia A
C. Hereditary hemolytic telangiectasia
D. Henoch-Scholein purpura

11. **A reliable screening test for platelet function is:**

A. CT
B. PT
C. Thrombin time
D. Clot retraction time

12. **Blood group antigens are:**

A. Carried by sex chromosomes
B. Attached to plasma proteins
C. Attached to Hemoglobin molecule
D. Found in saliva

13. **The greatest amount of CO_2 is transported in the blood as:**

A. RBC's
B. Bicarbonate ion
C. Plasma
D. All of the above

14. **The best screening test for hemophilia is:**

A. BT B. PT
C. PTT D. CT

15. **Thromboxane A2 is released mainly by the:**

A. Platelets
B. Vascular endothelium
C. Liver
D. Muscles

16. **Cyanosis is seen if the concentration of methaemoglobin is more than:**

A. 1.5 gm% B. 2.0 gm%
C. 3.0 gm% D. 4.0 gm%

17. **Half life of transfused platelets is:**

A. 4 hours B. 12 hours
C. 4 days D. 17 days

18. **In an adult man, there is about.......g hemoglobin in circulating blood.**

A. 350 B. 500
C. 900 D. 1000

19. **Increased activity of delta-amino lavullinic synthetase results in:**

A. Thalassemia
B. Sickle cell anaemia
C. Porphyria
D. Megaloblastic anaemia

20. **What does characterize function of platelets?**

A. From thrombus and release serotonin
B. Initiate and accelerate a lot formation
C. Contribute, possibly to integrity of capillary membrane
D. All of the above

21. **Which one of the following represents the most potentially dangerous situation?**

A. Rh positive mother with 2nd Rh-negative child
B. Rh negative mother with 2nd Rh-positive child
C. Rh positive mother with 1st Rh negative child
D. Rh- negative mother with 1st Rh positive child

22. **The absence of anti-A and anti-Rh agglutinins in plasma means the subject is:**

A. A positive or AP positive
B. A negative or AB negative
C. A positive, AP positive
D. Type O

23. The life span of the average erythrocyte in a newborn is:

A. 100 days
B. 120 days
C. 160 days
D. 8 months

24. The normal A/G ratio in blood is:

A. 5:1
B. 2:1
C. 1:2
D. 1:1

25. Which of the following statements about lymphocytes is incorrect?

A. Produced by thymus, red bone marrow, spleen and lymph nodes
B. Concentration falls in blood abruptly and immune reaction is disturbed after removal of thymus into plasma cells
C. Probably change into plasma cells
D. Constitute 20-40% of leukocytes

26. Which one of the following statements concerning monocyte is incorrect?

A. More common in blood than eosinophil and basophil
B. Produced in the adult by the bone marrow and lymph nodes
C. Unlike neutrophil
D. Is rich in lipase

27. A patient has a plasma concentration of HCO_3 of 13 mm/L and a plasma PCO_2 of 50 mm Hg. He has:

A. Compensated metabolic acidosis
B. Compensated respiratory acidosis
C. Respiratory acidosis and metabolic acidosis
D. Compensated respiratory alkalosis

28. The No. of O_2 molecules carried by on Hb molecule:

A. 1
B. 2
C. 4
D. 8

29. The No. of Fe atoms in one Hb molecule is:

A. 1
B. 2
C. 4
D. 8

30. Arneth Count is counting of:

A. Lymphocytes
B. Lobes in neutrophils
C. Granules in eosinophils
D. WBC in bone marrow

31. In vitro coagulation is initiated by factor:

A. XII
B. XI
C. X
D. VII

32. The best method for estimation of Hb concentration in blood is:

A. Acid haematin method
B. Alkali haematin method
C. Cyanmethaemoglobin method
D. Any of the above

33. Life of R.B.C. is:

A. 30 days
B. 90 days
C. 120 days
D. 160 days

34. Thrombosthenin is present in:

A. Plasma
B. Platelets
C. Neutrophils
D. RBC's

35. Hb is a good buffer because of:

A. Histidine residues
B. Protein nature
C. Acidic nature
D. Fe molecule

36. Christmas disease results to lack of which of the following factor of coagulation?

A. Factor V B. Factor VIII
C. Factor IX D. Factor X

37. Thrombosthenin is:

A. Coagulation factor
B. Contractile protein
C. A thrombosis promoting protein
D. A protein regulating platelet production

38. The cell membrane of human erythrocytes is more permeable to:

A. Cl- than K^+
B. K^+ than Na^+
C. K^+ than urea
D. Glucose than glycerol

39. The life span of platelets is:

A. 4 days B. 9-12 days
C. 20-30 days D. 90 days

40. Aggregation of platelets is inhibited by:

A. Ca^{++}
B. ADP
C. Thrombin
D. None of the above

41. Haemoglobin first appears in:

A. Early normoblast
B. Intermediate normoblast
C. Late normoblast
D. Pronormoblast

42. What does facilitate the conversion of profibrinolysin to fibrinolysin?

A. Tissue enzymes
B. Streptokinase
C. Urokinase
D. All of the above

43. Neutropenia is seen in all except:

A. Pernicious anaemia
B. Severe bacterial infection
C. Trauma
D. Bone marrow depression

44. MCHC (g/dl) is:

A. 7.5 B. 29
C. 34 D. 87

45. Stuart Prower factor is factor:

A. VIII B. IX
C. X D. XII

46. Factor used in the extrinsic pathway of blood coagulation is:

A. V B. VIII
C. Tissue factor III D. X

47. Respiratory alkalosis may be produced by:

A. Chronic obstructive pulmonary disease
B. Drugs causing respiratory depression
C. Hyperpnoea
D. Excessive renal bicarbonate absorption

48. What is wrong regarding factor VIII vWF?

A. Factor VIII is produced by liver
B. vWF is produced by endothelial cell
C. vWF prevents platelet adhesion with collagen
D. Factor VIII activates factor X

49. Hb E is formed due to replacement of glutamic acid at 26th position by..........

A. Glycine B. Lysine
C. Arginine D. Valine

50. The need for Vitamin B12 and folic acid in the formation of red blood cells is related primarily of their effects on:

A. Synthesis and release of erythropoietin from the kidney
B. Absorption of iron from the gut
C. DNA synthesis in Bone marrow
D. Hemoglobin formation in the red blood cell

51. Erythropoietin is increased in:

A. Blood loss B. High altitude
C. Exercise D. All of the above

52. Which one of the following statements regarding oxygenation and deoxygenation of haemoglobin (Hb) is correct?

A. Oxygenation Hb is a stronger acid when compared to deoxygenated Hb
B. Deoxygenated Hb is a stronger acid when compared to oxygenated Hb
C. The acidic characters of the oxygenated Hb and deoxygenated Hb are of the same magnitude
D. Since Hb is present inside the erythrocytes, its oxygenation or decarboxylation does not alter the acidic or basic character.

53. Platelets growth factor are synthesized by:

A. Glial cells B. Endothelium
C. Fibroblasts D. All of the above

54. Eosinophilia is caused by all except:

A. Stress B. Aspirin
C. PAN D. Ascariasis

55. The conversion of fibrinogen into fibrin occurs by:

A. Prothrombin B. Thrombin
C. Thrombophlebitis D. Platelets

56. What is the first important event in hemostasis following severe tissue injury?

A. Blood coagulation
B. Formation of a platelet plug
C. Vascular spasm
D. Formation of thromboplastin

57. When infection occurs a tissue, what type of white blood cells is first attracted from the blood into the tissue by the process of chemotaxis?

A. Neutrophils B. Monocytes
C. Eosinophils D. Basophils

58. What is the maximum concentration of hemoglobin normally found in red blood cells?

A. 5% B. 10%
C. 16% D. 20%
E. 34%

59. Mean corpuscular diameter (nm) is:

A. 4.1 B. 6.3
C. 7.2 D. 7.5

60. Cells with more than ....MCV/(fl) are called macrocytes.

A. 80 B. 87
C. 90 D. 95

61. Reticulocytes are stained with:

A. Methyl violet
B. Brilliant cresyl blue
C. Sudan black
D. Indigo carmine

62. In a person with type O blood, what type or types of agglutinins does he have in plasma?

A. None B. Alpha
C. Beta D. Alpha and beta

63. **Vitamin B 12 is essential for what aspect of blood cell reproduction?**

A. Formation of hemoglobin
B. Extrusion of the nucleus from the normoblasts
C. Formation of DNA
D. Activation of erythropoietin

64. **The most common site of haemopoiesis in Foetus is:**

A. Liver B. Spleen
C. Bone marrow D. Gut

65. **In anaemia, the concentration of 2,3 DPG is:**

A. Decreased B. Increased
C. a or b D. Not changed

66. **Alkali resistant Hb is:**

A. Hb A B. Hb A2
C. Hb F D. HbS

67. **Myoglobin bind with:**

A. 1 mol of oxygen per mol
B. 2 mol of oxygen per mol
C. 3 mol of oxygen per mol
D. 4 mol of oxygen per mol

68. **H^+ is more bound to:**

A. Deoxygenated hemoglobin
B. Oxygenated hemoglobin
C. Both a+b equally
D. Not related to oxygenation

69. **Haematocrit of venous blood is:**

A. 3% greater than arterial blood
B. 3 times greater than arterial blood
C. 3% less than arterial blood
D. 3 times less than arterial blood

70. **Haematocrit is ratio of:**

A. WBC to plasma
B. Platelets to plasma
C. RBC's to plasma
D. Total blood cells to plasma

71. **All are correct about potassium balance except:**

A. Most potassium is intracellular
B. Three quarter of the total body potassium is found in skeletal muscle
C. Intracellular potassium is released into extracellular space in response to severe injury to surgical stress
D. Acidosis leads to movement of potassium from extracellular to intracellular fluid compartment

72. **A shift of posture from supine to upright posture is associated with cardiovascular adjustments. Which of the following is NOT true in this context?**

A. Rise in central venous pressure
B. Rise in heart rate
C. Decrease in cardiac output
D. Decrease in stroke volume

73. **Shape of RBC is maintained by:**

A. Integrin B. Spectrin
C. Globin D. Ankyrin

74. **Cyanosis is caused by:**

A. Reduced Hb above 7.5 gm/dl
B. Met Hb above 1.5 g/dl
C. Sulph. Hb above 0.5 g/dl
D. All of the above

75. **Blood is non-Newtonian fluid because:**

A. Viscosity changes with velocity
B. Density changes with velocity
C. Density does not change with velocity
D. Viscosity does not change with velocity

76. Erythropoietin is secreted by A/E:

A. Hemangioblastoma
B. Hepatoma
C. Renal cell carcinoma
D. Adrenocortical tumours

77. Increased osmotic fragility is found in all except:

A. Spectrin deficiency
B. G-6PD deficiency
C. Hereditary hemolytic anemia
D. Sickle cell disease

78. A haematocrit of 41% in the sample of blood analysed means:

A. 41% of the blood volume is the plasma
B. 41% of the total blood volume is made up of plasma
C. 41% of the blood volume is the red blood cells
D. 41% of the total blood volume is made up of red and white blood cells and platelets

79. Clotting factor which is not formed by liver:

A. 10 B. 7
C. 8 D. 2

80. Glycophrin is seen in:

A. Enterocyte B. Erythrocyte
C. Lymphocyte D. Hepatocyte

81. Increase blood viscosity and slow circulation causes:

A. RBC Rouleux formation
B. Increase Plasma skimming
C. Increase number of RBC is capillaries
D. Increase WBC's count

82. The affinity of oxygen for Hb increased with fall in pH. This is called:

A. Bainbridge effect
B. Bohr effect
C. Haldane effect
D. Herring effect

EXPLANATORY ANSWERS OF BLOOD

1. **Ans. B:** Polycythemia is characterized by an increase in RBC count, making the blood viscous. This increases the peripheral resistance. (AK Jain 65)

2. **Ans. D:** Vit K is required for synthesis of factors II, VII, IX, X (2+7=9,10). (AK Jain 105,106)

3. **Ans. C:** Carbondioxide is transported as HCO_3-, carbaminohemoglobin and dissolved in plasma. (AK Jain 461)

4. **Ans. B:** Osmotic fragility is increased in hereditary spherocytosis and decreased in sickle cell anemia. (AK Jain 64)

5. **Ans. B:** Hemophilia is characterized by deficiency of factor VIII. (AK Jain 106)

6. **Ans. B:** Thalassemia is characterized by deficient alpha or beta chains. Fetal hemoglobin has alpha and gamma chains. (AK Jain 61)

7. **Ans. B:** Transferrin is the transport form of iron and ferritin is the storage form. (AK Jain 51, 283)

8. **Ans. C:** Cyanosis does not manifest in severe anemia because Hb < 5 gm%. (AK Jain 492-493)

9. **Ans. C:** Plasma is stored in the freezer with an acid citrate dextrose (ACD) buffer. (AK Jain 116)

10. **Ans. A:** Von Willebrand factor attaches factor VIII to platelets. Its deficiency leads to both increase in bleeding and clotting time. (AK Jain 94,102,106)

11. **Ans. D:** Thrombosthenin, platelet contractile proteins contract and help in clot retraction 48 hours after injury. Within 5-30 min clot retracts to 40% of its original volume. (AK Jain 96, 99)

12. **Ans. D:** The persons are called secretors (80%). ABO antigens are also found in organs like pancreas, kidney, urine, liver and lungs, testes, semen and amniotic fluid. (AK Jain 110)

13. **Ans. B:** 75% is in bicarbonate form, 18% is in carbamino compound, 7% is dissolved in plasma. (AK Jain 461)

14. **Ans. C:** Fresh frozen plasma or cryo-precipitates are given in Hemophilia. (AK Jain 105-107)

15. **Ans. A:** Thromboxane A2 promotes platelet aggregation and vasoconstriction. (AK Jain 96)

16. **Ans. A:** Cyanosis can be seen in areas where the skin is thin example mucus membrane of tongue, lips, ear lobes, nail beds, tip of nose. (AK Jain 492-493)

17. **Ans. C:** Life span of circulating platelets is 8-12 days. (AK Jain 96, 99)

18. **Ans. C:** Adult male Hb:14-18 gm% (Average 15.5 gm%). 5000 ml of blood will contain 750-900 gm of Hb. (AK Jain 58)

19. **Ans. C:** Synthesis of porphyrin ring of Hemoglobin is controlled by rate limiting enzyme delta aminolevulinic acid. (AK Jain 58, 59)

20. **Ans. D:** Platelets secrete 5-HT to cause vasoconstriction, adhere to collagen to form temporary hemostatic plug, lay the surface for deposition of fibrin for definitive hemostatic plug and help in clot retraction. (AK Jain 96, 99)

21. **Ans. B:** Injection of Anti D antibody within 48 hours of delivery of first baby prevents erythroblastosis fetalis. (AK Jain 78,113)

22. **Ans. C:** Landsteiner law states if agglutinins is absent, agglutinogen will be present. (AK Jain 111)

23. **Ans. A:** Life span can be determined by injecting radioactive iron. (AK Jain 64)

24. **Ans. B:** Normal A/G ratio is 1.7:1. It is reversed in liver diseases, nephrosis. (AK Jain 50, 51)

25. **Ans. B:** At puberty the thymus regresses. In children lymphocytes (60%) are more than neutrophils (40%) called *relative lymphocytosis*. (AK Jain 119)

26. **Ans. D:** Monocytes increase in tuberculosis and chronic bacterial infections. (AK Jain 88, 89)

27. **Ans. C:** Metabolic acidosis is characterized by a decrease in HCO_3^- ions secondary to increase in H^+ ions as in diabetes mellitus. Respiratory acidosis is characterized by decreased pulmonary ventilation which causes increased carbondioxide accumulation as in morphine administration. (AK Jain 478, 574, 576)

28. **Ans. C:** There are 4 haem to one molecule of haemoglobin, contains 4 iron atoms and can carry 4 molecules (8 atoms) of oxygen. (AK Jain 56)

29. **Ans. C:** Iron in the haem stays in the Fe^{++} state. (AK Jain 56, 57)

30. **Ans. B:** As the neutrophil grows old the nucleus becomes multilobed. (AK Jain 86, 89)

31. **Ans. A:** Factor XII is Hageman factor or glass factor that is activated by exposing to electronegatively charged surface like glass. (AK Jain 100,101)

32. **Ans. C:** The rods may fade over time in Sahli's haemoglobinometer and is subject to error.

33. **Ans. C:** RBC's are destroyed by tissue macrophage system. (AK Jain 64)

34. **Ans. B:** Thrombosthenin, platelet contractile proteins contract and help in clot retraction 48 hours after injury. (AK Jain 97,101,102)

35. **Ans. A:** 70% of buffer is provided by Hb. Pk value of Histidine (COO- and NH_3^+ terminal) is close to ph of 7.4. It is amphoteric in nature. (AK Jain 569)

36. **Ans. C:** Christmas disease is also called Hemophilia B and is due to congenital deficiency of factor IX. Clotting time is prolonged. (AK Jain 106)

37. **Ans. B:** Thrombosthenin, platelet contractile proteins contract and help in clot retraction 48 hours after injury. (AK Jain 97,101,102)

38. **Ans. B:** Cell membrane of RBC has a contractile layer of lipoprotein called "spectrin" that maintains the shape and flexibility. (AK Jain 63)

39. **Ans. B:** Life span can be studied by transfusing platelets labeled with ^{51}Cr or ^{32}P. (AK Jain 47, 94)

40. **Ans. D:** Prostacyclins inhibit platelet aggregation. ADP, Platelet activating factor help platelet aggregation. (AK Jain 94, 95)

41. **Ans. B:** The cytoplasm shows polychromatophilic staining at this stage. (AK Jain 70, 71)

42. **Ans. D:** These enzymes are fibrinolytic and can be used in the treatment of early MI and TIA. Urokinase is an enzyme produced by kidney cells. Streptokinase is a bacterial enzyme produced by streptococcus bacteria. Human TPA can be produced by DNA techniques. (AK Jain 104)

43. **Ans. C:** Neutropenia is seen in children, typhoid fever, viral infection and bone marrow depression. In trauma, surgery and burns after tissue destruction neutrophils increase in number. (AK Jain 86)

44. **Ans. C:** Mean corpuscular hemoglobin concentration (MCHC) is the concentration

of hemoglobin in one RBC (Hb/PCV). It equals 33 ± 3%. (AK Jain 66)

45. **Ans. C:** Factor X is also called auto-prothrombin C or Stuart prower factor. (AK Jain 100, 101)
46. **Ans. C:** Tissue thromboplastin (III), VII are the factors exclusive to extrinsic system. (AK Jain 100, 101)
47. **Ans. C:** Increase alveolar ventilation causes wash out of carbon dioxide and respiratory alkalosis. The causes are Hyperventilation at high altitude, voluntary or due to anxiety. (AK Jain 574, 575)
48. **Ans. C:** von Willebrand's factor plays an important role in platelet adhesion and regulates circulating level of factor VIII. (AK Jain 94,102,106)
49. **Ans. D:** HbE is not associated with sickling. In HbS at position 6 of beta chain one glutamic acid is replaced by valine. (AK Jain 59-60)
50. **Ans. C:** Within 6-9 hours of treatment with Vitamin B12 formation of nuclear DNA component promotes normoblastic reaction of the bone marrow. Folic acid also promotes the formation of nucleic acids. (AK Jain 72,73)
51. **Ans. D:** Hypoxia due to haemorrhage, high altitude, hormones like thyroxine, androgens increase erythropoietin. (AK Jain 72)
52. **Ans. B:** Oxyhemolobin is HbO_2. Deoxygenated or reduced Hb is Hb. This form is similar to carbaminohaemoglobin HBNHCOO. Hence more acidic than the oxygenated form. (AK Jain 57)
53. **Ans. D:** Platelet derived growth factor (PDGF) is also present in alpha granules of platelets. They stimulate wound healing and stimulates repair of the damaged vessel wall. (AK Jain 95, 96)
54. **Ans. A:** Eosinophilia is caused by parasitic infestation, e.g., **parasitic** infestation: worms, **allergic** conditions bronchial asthma, **skin** diseases (Remember : PAS). Eosinopenia is seen in stress and injection of ACTH. (AK Jain 87)
55. **Ans. B:** Thrombin (II), XIII (Fibrin stabilizing factor) and Calcium causes conversion of fibrinogen to fibrin. (AK Jain 101)
56. **Ans. C:** Haemostasis or cessation of bleeding is divided into Vasospasm, Platelet temporary hemostatic plug, fibrin clot definitive hemostatic plug and clot retraction. (AK Jain 98)
57. **Ans. A:** Neutrophils are the first line of defence. Monocytes form the second line of defence. (AK Jain 88, 89)
58. **Ans. E:** MCHC is never > 34% or hyperchromic as hemoglobin would precipitate out in the supersaturated solution of RBC. (AK Jain 66)
59. **Ans. D:** Microcytic anemia is seen in Iron deficiency. Megaloblastic anemia is seen in Vitamin B12 and folic acid deficiency. (AK Jain 77, 75)
60. **Ans. D:** Megaloblasts have MCV >110 fl. (AK Jain 75)
61. **Ans. B:** This is a form of supravital staining in which cells are stained while living. It takes two days from reticulocytes to become RBC. (AK Jain 70)
62. **Ans. D:** Blood group O were classically called Universal Donors, as they contain no agglutinogen. (AK Jain 110,111)
63. **Ans. C:** Within 6-9 hours of treatment with Vitamin B12 formation of nuclear DNA component promotes normoblastic reaction of the bone marrow. Folic acid also promotes the formation of nucleic acids. (AK Jain 72, 73)
64. **Ans. A:** In children erythropoiesis occurs in liver, spleen, all bones with red marrow.

In adults the sites of red marrow are end of long bones, skull, vertebrae, ribs, sternum and pelvis. (AK Jain 68)

65. **Ans. B:** In anaemia 2,3 DPG concentration increases making more oxygen available to the tissues. (AK Jain 74, 458)
66. **Ans. C:** This property is made use of in a photoelectric calorimetric method to estimate HbF in presence of Hb A.s (AK Jain 59, 60)
67. **Ans. A:** Myoglobin is specialized for sustained muscular contraction. It has only one heme group and does not show Bohr effect. (AK Jain 459)
68. **Ans. A:** Oxyhemolobin is HbO_2. Deoxygenated or reduced Hb is Hb. This form is similar to carbaminohaemoglobin HBNHCOO. Hence more acidic than the oxygenated form. (AK Jain 57)
69. **Ans. A:** The red blood cells are larger in venous blood due to chloride shift. Chloride moves inside the cell, as HCO_3^- moves out. Chloride imbibes water that makes the cell bigger. Consequently hematocrit is more in venous blood. (AK Jain 47, s464)
70. **Ans. C:** Haematocrit is called Volume of Packed red blood cells (VPRBC) as it does not include the volume of white blood cells and platelets. Its value is 45%. (AK Jain 47)
71. **Ans. D:** In acidosis the excess H^+ moves into the cell and K+ moves out to balance the electrical gradient. This principle is used in treatment of hyperkalemia when insulin is given with dextrose drip to cause K+ to move into the cell and H+ out. (AK Jain 543)
72. **Ans. A:** A change in supine to upright posture is associated with an increase in sympathetic drive and venous pooling. The heart rate consequently rises but stroke volume and cardiac output fall. Central venous pressure in the jugulars is maintained at -5 to -7 mm Hg. (AK Jain 408)
73. **Ans. B:** Spectrin is absent from the red blood cell membrane in hereditary spherocytosis. This leads to increased fragility and easy destruction of the RBC's. The condition is called hemolytic anemia. (AK Jain 63)
74. **Ans. D:** Cyanosis or blue discolouration of mucous membrane is an index of hypoxia or deceased oxygen at the tissue level. It may occur in stagnant hypoxia, hypoxic hypoxia. Methaemoglobinemia may be treated by reducing Fe+++ by methylene blue. Severe anemic hypoxia < 5 gm% can never result in cyanosis (reduced Hb > 5 gm%). (AK Jain 492-493)
75. **Ans. A:** Reynold number is an index of velocity of blood. At high viscosity the flow is streamlined, at lower viscosity higher flow rates or turbulence occur. (AK Jain 331)
76. **Ans. D:** Erythropoietin causes erythropoiesis in 3-7 days after secretion from kidneys in response to hypoxia. The Ep may also be secreted from tumors of vascular tissue, kidney and liver. (AK Jain 72)
77. **Ans. D:** In sickle cell anemia the cell is small in size, and can imbibe more water. The osmotic fragility of these cells is thus low. They are however mechanically fragile. In the other conditions the RBC are readily broken down; hemolytic anemia and are osmotically fragile. (AK Jain 61)
78. **Ans. C:** Haematocrit is called Volume of Packed red blood cells (VPRBC) as it does not include the volume of white blood cells and platelets. Its value is 41% in this case. (AK Jain 47)
79. **Ans. C:** Factors 2,7,9,10 are carboxylated in the liver by Vit K. 8 comes from endothelial cells. (AK Jain 106)
80. **Ans. B:** Spectrins, ankyrins and glycophorins are membrane cytoskeletal proteins providing for shape and flexible to the RBC. (AK Jain 63)

81. **Ans. A:** Rouleax are stacks of RBC like coins one on top of the other. Fibrinogen, increase in viscocity promotes rouleax formation. (AK Jain 54)

82. **Ans. B:** Increase in basal low heart rate on infusing saline is called Bain bridge effect. Loading of CO_2 causing unloading of O_2 at tissue level is called Haldane effect. Herring Breur reflex is the prolongation of duration of expiration after increased inflation. This protects the lung from hyperinflation. (AK Jain 348, 463, 470)

CHAPTER 7

Gastrointestinal System (GIT)

What is Important in GIT?

Functional Types of Movements, Digestion of Food, Important Local Hormones

1. The only sugar normally absorbed by the intestine against a concentration gradient is:

A. Xylose
B. Mannose
C. Glucose
D. Ribose

2. Surface protection is given by following except:

A. Mucin
B. IgA
C. Pepsin
D. All of the above

3. In distal ileum resection, following are seen except:

A. B12 deficiency
B. Fe deficiency
C. Decrease absorption of bile salts
D. None

4. Surgical removal of about 90% of the ileum and jejunum tends to cause all, except:

A. An increase in fat content of stool
B. Demineralisation of bones
C. A fall in extracellular fluid volume
D. Anaemia

5. All is true for cells of liver, except:

A. Are important site for synthesis of plasma albumin
B. Are the only important site for synthesis of plasma globulins
C. Can store Vitamin B12
D. Release glucose when blood glucose level tends to fall below normal

6. The duodenum secretes a hormone which has following effects except:

A. Exerts trophic action in pancreas
B. Increases gastric motility
C. Causes gallbladder to contract and sphincter to relax
D. Leads to meager flow of pancreatic juice rich in enzymes

7. Two basic types of electrical waves in smooth muscle of the gastrointestinal tract are:

A. Fast waves and spikes
B. Short and long spikes

C. Slow waves and spikes
D. Slow waves and fast waves

8. **The usual stimulus of peristalsis is:**
A. Distention
B. Sympathetic stimulation
C. Acid chyme
D. Alkaline chime

9. **The principal function of the gastro-esophageal sphincter is:**
A. To allow stomach acid into the esophagus
B. To maintain food in the esophagus for digestion
C. To prevent reflux of stomach contents
D. Non existent

10. **Which of the following is not present in the pancreatic juice?**
A. Aminopeptidase B. Elastase
C. Colipase D. Ribonuclease

11. **Which converts chymotrypsinogen to chymotrypsin?**
A. Trypsin B. Low pH
C. Chymosin D. Pepsinogen

12. **Ingestion of a meal containing only protein would result in:**
A. Hypoglycemia
B. Increased insulin release
C. Decreased insulin release
D. Decreased hepatic glycogen

13. **The three phases of gastric secretion are:**
A. First, Second and Third
B. Cephalic, gastric and intestinal
C. Ptyalin, gastrin and intestinal
D. Gastric, intestinal, colonic

14. **Hydrochloric acid is secreted by the:**
A. Paneth cells B. Goblet cells
C. Chief cells D. Parietal cells

15. **Sympathectomy ..... mucus secretion by the intestine.**
A. Decreases B. Increases
C. Has no effect D. A or B

16. **Duodenal mucosa is protected from the action of acid and pepsin by:**
A. Reduced secretion of bicarbonate
B. Secretion of Brunner's glands
C. Hyperplasia of duodenal mucosa
D. Stimulation of sympathetics

Match the following:
A. Myentric reflex
B. Gastrocolic reflex
C. Mass movement
D. Segmentation
E. Law of intestine

17. **Local, non propagated contraction and relaxation of the intestine**

18. **Single, vigorous peristaltic contraction and relaxation of the intestine**

19. **A dilatation of intestinal lumen causes contraction above and relaxation of the intestine**

20. **Peristalsis travels from the oral to the aboral end of the intestine**

21. **Ingestion of food causes an increase in motility of large intestine**

Match the following:
A. Cholagogue
B. Cholerectic

C. Hydrocholerectic
D. Cholecystokinin

22. Increases bile flow by contracting gall-bladder

23. Increases the output of bile from liver

24. Increases flow of bile into intestine

25. Increases the volume of bile but not necessarily the amount of bile solid

26. An adult human pancreas has about:

A. 1000-2000 islets
B. 100,000-200,000 islets
C. 250,000-750,000 islets
D. Above 1000,000 islets

27. The mechanism which causes maximum gastric secretion is:

A. Cholinergic receptor stimulation
B. H2 receptor stimulation
C. Neurogenic
D. Na K ATPase pump

28. The normal basal acid output is…mmol/hour.

A. 2-3 B. 5-10
C. 15-20 D. 20-25

29. The normal portal venous pressure is…..mm Hg.

A. 4-6 B. 8-12
C. 25-30 D. 12-16

30. Vagal stimulation following intake of food does not affect secretion of:

A. Pancreas
B. Gastric mucosa
C. Gallbladder
D. Parotid

31. Gastric emptying is decreased by all of the following except:

A. Distention of duodenum
B. Alkaline pH in duodenum
C. Fatty meal
D. Hyperosmolarity in duodenum

32. The following are hormones secreted locally in gut except:

A. Gastrin
B. Enterogastrone
C. Secretin
D. None of the above

33. False about Pancreatic secretion is:

A. 1 L/day
B. Osmolarity ½ of plasma
C. Secretin produces HCO_3 rich
D. Pancreozymin enzyme rich

34. Cation more in gastric secretion than in blood is:

A. Sodium B. Potassium
C. Calcium D. Magnesium

35. Calcium absorption is controlled by:

A. Vitamin
B. Parathormone
C. Both
D. None of the above

36. Pepsinogen I is secreted from:

A. Parietal cells
B. Chief cells
C. G-cells
D. Mucous cells

37. Which of the following is not required for calcium absorption?

A. Parathyroid hormone

B. Calcitonin
C. Vitamin D
D. Bile salts

38. Prolonged vomiting may result in:
A. Metabolic acidosis
B. Metabolic alkalosis
C. Respiratory acidosis
D. Respiratory alkalosis

39. Salivary amylase digests starch in:
A. Mouth B. Stomach
C. Duodenum D. Jejunum

40. Of total hepatic blood flow, hepatic artery supplies...%.
A. 15-20 B. 25-30
C. 35-50 D. 50-65

41. Liver has the maximum O_2 consumption (51 ml/min), the next organ to have the maximum O_2 (ml/min) is:
A. Heart B. Brain
C. Skeletal muscle D. Kidney

42. Lipase is not present in:
A. Saliva
B. Pancreatic juice
C. Succus entericus
D. Gastric juice

43. All of the following are sources of Liver glycogen except:
A. Glycerol B. Fructose
C. Lactic acid D. Triglycerides

44. Iron is absorbed almost entirely in:
A. Stomach B. Duodenum
C. Jejunum D. Ileum

45. The first part of test meal reaches the caecum in about....hours, the hepatic flexure in....hours, the splenic flexure in...hours and sigmoid colon in.... hours.
A. 4,6,9,12 B. 6,9,12,16
C. 2,4,6,8 D. 2,6,8,12

46. One of the following is not a constituent of saliva:
A. Glucose B. Bicarbonate
C. Lysozyme D. Phosphate

47. Gastrocolic reflex causes:
A. Pendular movement
B. Mass peristalsis
C. Colonic disease
D. All of the above

48. Failure to absorb Vitamin B12 from the gastrointestinal tract results in a syndrome called:
A. Pernicious anemia
B. Hemolytic anemia
C. Polycythemia
D. Thallesemia

49. After absorption, iron in blood is:
A. Apoferritin B. Ferritin
C. Transferrin D. Cerruloplasmin

50. Maximum absorption of bile occurs at:
A. Jejunum B. Duodenum
C. Ileum D. Colon

51. Which of the following is fastest to be absorbed from stomach?
A. Carbohydrates B. Proteins
C. Fats D. Water

52. The type of taste is most sensitive to minute concentrations of the substance to be tasted is:
A. The sour taste B. The salty taste
C. The sweet taste D. The bitter taste

53. Intestinal juice contains:

A. Enzymes responding to vagal activity
B. Saccharidase
C. Potassium equal in concentration to extracellular fluid
D. A substance which activates trypsinogen activity

54. Exocrine secretion of pancrease is controlled by:

A. Secretin
B. Cholecystokinin
C. N-benzyaol-L-tytesyl amino benzoic acid
D. All of the above

55. True about Gastrin:

A. Marked secretion of pepsinogen
B. Decreased gastric motility
C. Acid stimulates gastrin secretion
D. Is a polypeptide

56. False about ileum and jejunal resection:

A. Results in pale bulky stools
B. Osteomalacia
C. Steatorrhea
D. Rise in prothrombin time

57. Hepatic failure results in:

A. Low A:G ratio
B. High A:G ratio
C. High serum albumin
D. Jaundice always

58, There are about ....acini in human liver.

A. 10,000 B. 1 lac
C. 10 lacs D. 50 lacs

59. Daily secretions of gastrointestinal tract amount to:

A. 8000 ml B. 4000 ml
C. 2000 ml D. 2 to 4 liters

60. Process of normal swallowing involves all except:

A. Vocal cords approximation
B. Soft palate elevation
C. Palatopharyngeal folds
D. Tracheal valves

61. Total gastrectomy may lead to:

A. Indigestion
B. Severe anemia
C. Giddiness
D. Dizziness, Pallor and swelling after meals

62. Water absorption is mainly a function of:

A. Colon B. Intestine
C. Stomach D. Liver

63. Sphincter of Oddi is located in:

A. Gastrium
B. Urinary bladder
C. Biliary system
D. Central nervous system

64. The most important stimulus for secretion of secretin is:

A. Vagal stimulation
B. Mechanical duodenal distention
C. Acidic chyme reaching duodenum
D. Fat reaching the duodenum

65. Gastric secretion is not influenced by:

A. Diet
B. Gastrin
C. Secretin
D. Cholecystokinin
E. None of the above

66. **Pancreatic juice rich in water and electrolytes but poor in enzymes is secreted in response to:**

A. Pancreatozymin
B. Cholecystokinin
C. Secretin
D. Proteins

67. **Vitamin B12 is absorbed from:**

A. Jejunum B. Proximal ileum
C. Terminal ileum D. Stomach

68. **In severe diarrhoea:**

A. Serum K+ level declines
B. Intravenous infusion should be given rapidly
C. Blood pressure declines and pulse rate increases
D. All of the above

69. **Cephalic phase of gastric secretion is mediated by:**

A. Neurohormones
B. Parasympathetic
C. Sympathetic
D. Gastrin

70. **A large greasy smelly stool usually indicates failure of digestion of:**

A. Carbohydrates B. Fats
C. Proteins D. Peptones

71. **The absence of lactase in the intestine would cause failure to digest completely:**

A. Steak B. Beer
C. Milk D. Peptones

72. **Failure to absorb bile salts in the distal ileum causes:**

A. Constipation B. No effect
C. Diarrhea D. Dysentry

73. **The hormone generally considered to be the major stimulus for enzyme secretion by the pancreas is:**

A. Cholecystokinin B. Secretin
C. Trypsin D. Gastrin

74. **Stored fat is usually transported from one part of the body to another part in the form of:**

A. Triglycerides B. Free fatty acids
C. Glycerol D. Neutral fat

75. **When excess amounts of carbohydrates or proteins are consumed, they are stored in the body as:**

A. Glucose B. Glycogen
C. Protein D. Triglycerides

76. **In which of the following situations is the secretion of saliva increased?**

A. When the touch receptors in the mouth are stimulated
B. Just before vomiting
C. When bitter food is placed in the tongue
D. All of the above

77. **Saliva differs from plasma in:**

A. Hypotonicity
B. HCO_3- concentration
C. Protease enzyme
D. Aldosterone decreases

78. **Maximum Na + concentration is found in:**

A. Pancreatic juice B. Gastric juice
C. Bile juice D. Intestinal juice

79. **Following are transitory movements of intestine:**

A. Peristalsis
B. Segmentation

C. Antiperistalsis

D. Mass peristalsis

80. Peristalsis may be initiated by or effected by all of the following except:

A. Inhibitors of striated contraction

B. The myentric plexus

C. Irritation of mucous

D. The composition of chime

81. An average 70 years man has .... kg glycogen in liver.

A. 0
B. 0.4
C. 0.8
D. 1.0

EXPLANATORY ANSWERS OF GIT

1. **Ans. C:** Glucose is the chief energy source, readily assimilated. Its absorption thus occurs actively against concentration gradient via sodium dependent glucose transporter (SGLT 1, Na+-glucose cotransporter) into the intestinal cell and then into the interstitium by simple diffusion or facilitated diffusion. (Ganong 430)
2. **Ans. C:** Peptic ulcer results when an imbalance between mucin and HCl occurs. IgA is protective and is found in body secretions. Pepsin serves to digest protein in milk, dals, meat. (Ganong 447)
3. **Ans. B:** Bile salts and Vitamin B12 are absorbed in the distal ileum, by enterohepatic circulation and intrinsic factor respectively. Most of the iron is absorbed in the upper intestine. (Ganong 436)
4. **Ans. C:** Water absorption primarily occurs in the large intestine. Bile salts and Vitamin B12 are absorbed in the distal ileum. Emulsification of fat is hampered that results in fatty stools (Steatorrhea). Most of the iron is absorbed in the upper intestine. Deficiency leads to anemia. (Ganong 433, 436)
5. **Ans. B:** Plasma immunoglobulins are synthesized by B lympocytes. Functions of liver are fomation of bile, metabolism of glucose, inactivation of toxins, providing immunity, synthesise plasma proteins. (Ganong 455, 475)
6. **Ans. B:** Cholecystokinin–Pancreozymin is released by fatty acids and amino acids in duodenum. It inhibits gastric motility. The other actions along with gastrin stimulates glucagons secretion. Prevents reflux of food in the stomach, by contracting the pyloric sphincter. (Ganong 454)
7. **Ans. C:** The gastric slow wave or basic electric rhythm (BER) is a wave of depolarization that proceeds from the circular muscle of the fundus of the stomach to the pylorus approximately every 20 seconds. It plays a major role in gastric emptying. (Ganong 449) The contractions of the small intestine are coordinated by small bowel slow wave. The direction is caudally at 12/min in the jejunum to about 9/min in the ileum. (Ganong 461)
8. **Ans. A:** Peristalsis helps move the contents from one part of the small or large intestine to the other like the squeezing of the toothpaste from the tube. (Ganong 461)
9. **Ans. C:** Achalasia cardia is a condition when food acculmulates in the lower esophagus and the organ becomes massively dilated. The opposite condition is lower esophagal incompetence, which cannot prevent reflux of stomach contents and results in heartburn and esophagitis. H_2 blockers or omeprazole or fundoplication (making a fold of gastric tissue) can be given. (Ganong 446)
10. **Ans. A:** Pancreatic juice has the following enzymes trypsinogen, chymotrypsinogen, proelastase, procarboxypeptidases. (Ganong 453)
11. **Ans. A:** Trypsinogen converts chymotrypsinogen into chymotrypsin that digests proteins. It also activates phospholipase A_2 that forms lysolecithin that damages cell membranes. It is not possible to operate on the pancrease (autocatalytic chain reaction). (Ganong 453)
12. **Ans. C:** Amino acids leucine, arginine are insulin and glucagons stimulators. Insulin is an anabolic hormone, building body protein. Protein diet will inhibit insulin release. (Ganong 314)

13. **Ans. B:** The sight, smell and thought of food increases gastric secretion (Cephalic). Food in stomach increases gastric secretion by mechanical distention. (Gastric). Duodenal chyme inhibits gastric secretion (Intestinal). (Ganong 450)
14. **Ans. D:** Hydrochloric acid is secreted by H+K+ ATPase in parietal cells. (Ganong 448)
15. **Ans. B:** Parasympahetic function increases gastric secretion and motility. Vagotomy however does not abolish the secretory response to local stimuli. (Ganong 449)
16. **Ans. B:** Mucus is secreted by Brunner's glands in duodenum and by characteristic goblet cells in mucosa of small and large intestine. (Ganong 460)
17. **Ans. D:** Segmentation helps in mixing the food and increase surface for absorption of chyme. It is similar to the wringing of a towel as ring like contractions appear and disappear at regular intervals.(Ganong 510)
18. **Ans. C:** Contractions of smooth muscle over large confluent areas of the colon are called mass peristalsis. They move material from one portion of the colon to the other. (Ganong 512)
19. **Ans. A:** Myentric plexus or Auerbach's plexus are between outer longitudinal and middle circular layers. Myentric plexus help in peristalsis or movement of chime towards The rectum. (Ganong 512)
20. **Ans. E:** The electrical activity is from oral to aboral, even if the individual stands on his Head (Shirshasana). The activity is basal electrical rhythm, migrating motor complex. (Ganong 510)
21. **Ans. B:** The gastrocolic reflex is presumably a vagal reflex, as food leaves the stomach the cecum relaxes and the passage of the chyme through ileocaecal valve increases. Gastrocolic reflex is characteristic when a baby drinks milk and has diarrhea or a man who needs to drink tea in the morning before the toilet. (Ganong 512)
22. **Ans. D:** Fatty acids and amino acids in duodenum release CCK, which cause gall-bladder contraction. (Ganong 502)
23. **Ans. B:** Substances increasing secretion of bile are called choleretics, e.g., Secretin, Bile salts. (Ganong 502)
24. **Ans. A:** Substances that cause contraction of gallbladder are called cholagogues, e.g., CCK.
25. **Ans. C:** % of bile solids in hepatic bile is 2-4% and bile salts 10-20% mmol/l as compared to gallbladder bile 10-12% solids and 50-200 mmol/L bile salts. The production of bile is increased by stimulation of vagus nerves, hormone secretin and bile salts. (Ganong 507)
26. **Ans. C:** Acinar cells secreting pancreatic juice resemble salivary glands as the contain Zymogen granules. (Ganong 501)
27. **Ans. B:** Acid secretion is increased by secretion by the action of acetylcholine on M_3 Muscarinic receptors, gastrin, histamine and PGE_2. They act to increase activity of H^+K^+ ATPase. (Ganong 497)
28. **Ans. B:** Cephalic influences (sight, smell, thought of food) stimulates gastric secretion. These are responsible for one third to one half of the acid secreted in response to a normal meal. (Ganong 498)
29. **Ans. B:** Portal venous pressure is about 10 mm Hg. Hepatic venous pressure is 5 mm Hg. Mean pressure in hepatic artery in sinusoids is 90 mm Hg. (Ganong 617)
30. **Ans. D:** Parotid gland receives nerve supply from auriculotempoal nerve. Food in mouth causes reflex secretion of saliva and so does stimulation of vagal afferent fibers at gastric end of esophagus.(Ganong 493)

31. **Ans. B:** Factors that increase gastric emptying include hunger, happy attitude, light exercise. Factors decreasing emptying include depression, pain, violent exercise, fear, proteins like meat, milk or lassi.

32. **Ans. D:** Gastrin is produced by cells called G cells. Secretin is secreted by S cells of Duodenum. Enterogastrone inhibits gastrin secretion and motility (Polypeptide YY). (Ganong 489, 490, 491)

33. **Ans. B:** Pancreatic secretion about 1500 ml/day. It is alkaline and high HCO_3^- content (approx 113 meq/l versus 24 meq/l plasma). Secretion produces juice rich in HCO_3^-, CCK acts on acinar cells to produce enzymes. Anions are Cl-, HPO_4^-, SO_4^-. (Ganong 496)

34. **Ans. A:** Cations in gastric juice are Na^+, K+, Mg++, H+, pH (approximately 1.0).

35. **Ans. C:** Vitamin D increases calcium and phosphorus in blood. Parathormone is the major hormone that causes decrease in calcium and increase in phosphorus in blood. Remodelling of bone by hormone parathormone results in formation of a new skeleton in seven years! Calcitonin deceases or tone down the level of calcium and phosphorus. (Ganong 391, 394)

36. **Ans. B:** Chief cells secrete pepsinogen, the inactive precursor of pepsin in gastric juice contains zymogen granules. Parietal cells secrete HCl.(Ganong 496)

37. **Ans. B:** The role of calcitonin is responsible for decreasing postprandial hyperglycemia. Calcitonin also may be protective to the mother during pregnancy when the fetal bones are being formed. (Ganong 398)

38. **Ans. B:** In metabolic alkalosis the plasma HCO_3^- level and pH rise. HCl extruded from the stomach leads to alkalosis.(Ganong 739)

39. **Ans. A:** Salivary amylase or ptyalin acts at pH 6.0-8.0 to digest starch. It gets deactivated at pH < 4.5. Salivary α amylase hydrolyses 1:4 α linkages, producing α-limit dextrins, maltotriose and maltose. Pancreatic α amylase has a similar action on starch in duodenum. (Ganong 472)

40. **Ans. B:** The liver receives about 1000 ml/min, from portal vein and 400 ml/min from hepatic artery. (Ganong 427)

41. **Ans. C:** Oxygen consumption of skeletal muscle is 50 ml/min, Brain 46 ml/min, Heart 29 ml/min and kidneys 18 ml/min. (Ganong 615t)

42. **Ans. C:** Lipase causes triglycerides to form fatty acids plus 1,2 diacylglycerol. (Ganong 472)

43. **Ans. C:** Glycogen is synthesized by glycogen synthase. Glycogen is a branched glucose polymer with two types of glycoside linkages 1:4 α and 1:6 α linkages. (Ganong 292)

44. **Ans. B:** Iron in the diet is Fe+++ and absorbed is Fe++. Fe is absorbed in duodenum via transporters ferroprotein 1 and hephaestin 1. (Ganong 481)

45. **Ans. A:** The first part of test meal reaches caecum in 4 hours and all undigested portions enter the colon in 8 or 9 hours. The test meal reaches the hepatic flexure in 6 hours, splenic flexure 9 hours and pelvic colon in 12 hours. From pelvic colon to anus transport is much slower. (Ganong 512)

46. **Ans. A:** Saliva contains lingual lipase, salivary amylase, mucins, Ig A, lysozyme, praline rich proteins, Na^+, K^+, Cl^- and HCO_3^-. (Ganong 492)

47. **Ans. B:** When food leaves the stomach the cecum relaxes and the passage of chime through the ileocaecal valve increases (gastroileal reflex). This is a vagal reflex. (Ganong 512)

48. **Ans. A:** Pernicious anemia is also called Addison's crisis. Totally gastrectomized patients develop intrinsic factor deficiency

and iron deficiency anemia that must be circumvented by parenteral injection of cyanocobalamin. (Ganong 500)

49. **Ans. C:** Transport of Iron is in Transferrin form. Ferritin is the storage form. Ferritin molecules in lysosomal membranes are called haemosiderin. Cerruloplasmin transports copper (Wilson's disease). (Ganong 482)

50. **Ans. C:** 90-95% of bile salts are absorbed from the terminal ileum by an extremely efficient Na+ - bile salt cotransporter powered by Na+ K+ ATPase (Enterohepatic circulation). (Ganong 505)

51. **Ans. D:** Food rich in carbohydrate leaves stomach in a few hours. Protein rich food leaves more slowly, and emptying after a meal containing fat is slowest. (Ganong 499)

52. **Ans. D:** Sweet taste is produced due to glucose. Salty due to Na+ ions. Sour taste due to H^+ ions. Bitter is a complex sensation. Strychnine hydrochloride stimulates bitter taste at threshold concentration of 1.6 μmol/l. Glucose stimulates sweet at 80,000 μmol/l. HCl sour at 100 μmol/l and NaCl salty at 2000 μmol/l. (Ganong 193)

53. **Ans. D:** Trypsinogen is converted to the active enzyme trypsin by the brush border enzyme enteropeptidase (Enterokinase) when pancreatic juice enters duodenum. (Ganong 502)

54. **Ans. D:** Secretin causes increase in bicarbonate, low in enzymes. CCK causes increase in enzymes, but low in volume. Acetylcoline has a similar action in pancreas. (Ganong 502)

55. **Ans. D:** Gastrin is a polypeptide hormone that shows macroheterogeneity (different lengths of peptide chains) and microheterogeneity (difference in single amino acid residue). Distension, Protein stimulates secretion. Acid, somatostatin inhibits secretion. Functions of gastrin are to stimulate gastric motility, insulin secretion, gastric acid and pepsin secretion. (Ganong 488, 489)

56. **Ans. D:** Resection of ileum prevents absorption of bile salts, that leads to deficient fat absorption. Other complications include hypocalcemia (osteomalacia), arthritis, hyperuricemia and possibly fatty infiltration of liver, followed by cirrhosis. (Ganong 511)

57. **Ans. A:** Albumin is synthesized in the liver. Globulin is synthesized by cells in plasma. Hepatic failure decreases the level of albumin. A/G ratio decreases. (Ganong 543, 504)

58. **Ans. B:** One acinus consists of a central vein, portal space containing branches of bile duct, portal vein and hepatic artery. (Ganong 504)

59. **Ans. A:** Total endogenous secretions from salivary glands, stomach, bile, pancreas, intestine is 9000 ml, 8800 ml is reabsorbed in jejunum, ileum and colon. Balance in stool is 200 ml. (Ganong 480)

60. **Ans. D:** Swallowing is initiated by the voluntary action of collecting the oral contents on the tongue and propelling them backward into the pharynx (oral phase). This starts a wave of involuntary contraction in the pharyngeal muscles pushing the material in esophagus. Inhibition of respiration and glottic closure occurs (pharyngeal phase). Peristaltic waves push the food into the stomach at the rate of 4 cm/sec (esophageal phase). (Ganong 493)

61. **Ans. A:** Totally gastrecomized patients develop intrinsic factor deficiency and iron deficiency anemia that must be circumvented by parenteral injection of cyanocobalamine. Protein digestion is normal in absence of pepsin. The patient must eat frequently. Weakness, dizziness and sweating after meals due to hypoglycemia is the picture

in "dumping syndrome" where portions of stomach have been removed. (Ganong 500)

62. **Ans. B:** The absorptive capacity of mucosa of large intestine is great. Na^+ is actively transported out of the colon, and water follows along the osmotic gradient thus generated. (Ganong 512)

63. **Ans. C:** In normal individuals, bile flows into the gallbladder when sphincter of Oddi is closed. In the gallbladder, the bile is concentrated by absorption of water. The common bile duct enters the duodenum papillae. Its orifice is surrounded by the sphincter of Oddi, that unites with the pancreatic duct before entering the duodenum. (Ganong 503, 507)

64. **Ans. C:** Secretin increases secretion of bicarbonate by duct cells of pancreas and biliary tract. Its secretion is increased by production of protein digestion and by acid bathing mucosa of upper small intestine. (Ganong 490)

65. **Ans. E:** Mechanisms that enhance motility are hunger, happy attitude, light exercise like walking, carbohydrate rich diet. Mechanisms that decrease motility are depression, fear, proteins, milk. (Ganong 450)

66. **Ans. C:** Fatty acids and amino acids in duodenum release CCK, which cause gall-bladder contraction.

67. **Ans. C:** Ileal resection results in Vitamin B12 deficiency and megaloblastic anemia.

68. **Ans. D:** The sight, smell and thought of food increases gastric secretion (Cephalic). Food in stomach increases gastric secretion by mechanical distention (Gastric). Duodenal chyme inhibits gastric secretion (Intestinal). (Ganong 450)

69. **Ans. B:** Cephalic phase of gastric secretion is mediated by vagus nerve in which the mere thought, sight, smell of food increases secretion. (Ganong 450)

70. **Ans. B:** Resection of ileum prevents absorption of bile salts, that leads to deficient fat absorption causing Steatorrhea. (Ganong 511)

71. **Ans. C:** Old people with deficiency of lactase have difficulty in digesting milk, digesting curds, milk and icecream.

72. **Ans. C:** Resection of ileum prevents absorption of bile salts, that leads to deficient fat absorption causing Steatorrhea. (Ganong 511)

73. **Ans. A:** Fatty acids and amino acids in duodenum release CCK, which cause gall-bladder contraction. Secretion produces juice rich in HCO_3^-, CCK acts on acinar cells to produce enzymes. (Ganong 502)

74. **Ans. B:** Free fatty acids are provided to fat cells and other tissues by chlyomicrons and VLDL. (Ganong 278)

75. **Ans. D:** Triglycerides are free fatty acids and glycerol, found in adipose tissue. (Ganong 278)

76. **Ans. D:** Xerostomia is deficiency of salivary secretion, have higher incidence of dental caries. (Ganong 445)

77. **Ans. D:** Saliva secreted in the acini is isotonic with the concentrations of Na^+, K^+, and HCO_3^-. Aldosterone increases the K^+ concentration and reduces the Na^+. (Ganong 445)

78. **Ans. C:** Alkaline bile has sodium and potassium salts of glycocholic and taurocholic acid. (Ganong 456)

79. **Ans. B:** Motility of small intestine includes peristalsis, segmental movements and peristalsis rush. (Ganong 461)

80. **Ans. A:** Mechanisms that enhance motility are hunger, happy attitude, light exercise like walking, carbohydrate rich diet. Mechanisms that decrease motility are depression, fear, proteins, milk. (Ganong 450)

81. **Ans. B:** During exercise the source of intracellular glucose is glycogen, the carbohydrate polymer that is abundant in liver and skeletal muscle. (Ganong 63)

CHAPTER 8

Respiration

What is Important in Lungs?

Pulmonary Function Tests (Various Capacities) and Effect of Common Diseases on Them, Transport of Gases (O_2, CO_2), Regulation of Respiration

1. **Alveolar ventilation (l/min) at rest is:**
   A. 3 B. 4.2
   C. 6 D. 125
2. **Surfactant is decreased or absent in:**
   A. Emphysema
   B. Bronchial asthma
   C. Respiratory distress syndrome in children (RDS)
   D. RDS in adults
3. **CO_2 enters capillaries by:**
   A. Diffusion
   B. Permeation
   C. Osmosis
   D. Active transport
4. **Carbonmonoxide is released in lungs from:**
   A. Iron of heme molecule
   B. Plasma
   C. Transferrin
   D. Plasma
5. **Effort during normal respiration is done for purpose:**
   A. Lung elasticity
   B. Respiratory air passages
   C. Alveolar air spaces
   D. Creating negative pleural pressure
6. **CO_2 influences respiration by acting at:**
   A. Cerebrum
   B. Carotid body
   C. Whole of medulla
   D. Respiratory centre
7. **Maximum voluntary ventilation (L/min) is:**
   A. 90-120 B. 125-170
   C. 170-210 D. 210-250
8. **An increase in ventilation occurs in all except:**
   A. Decreased Plasma HCO_3^-
   B. Decreased pH of CSF
   C. Increased Blood adrenaline
   D. None of the above
9. **A patient respiring 21/min (Pulmonary ventilation) and has respiratory rate of 20/min. Which of the following is true?**

A. Doing exercise
B. Decreased pH of CSF
C. Cheyne-Stokes breathing
D. Respiring in dead space

10. A person ascends to 12,000 feet, develops acute breathlessness, this is due to:

A. Decreased pulmonary blood flow
B. Carbon dioxide washout
C. Decreased hypoxic stimulation of respiration
D. Mechanical interference of thorax

11. The most important substance controlling alveolar ventilation:

A. Oxygen
B. Carbon dioxide
C. Water
D. None of the above

Match the following:

A. 3000 ml B. 4600 ml
C. 500 ml D. 3500 ml

12. Tidal volume

13. Inspiratory reserve volume

14. Vital capacity

15. Inspiratory capacity

16. The diffusing capacity for carbon dioxide compared to that for oxygen is:

A. 20 times B. 10 times
C. 5 times D. 2 times

17. Destruction of lung tissue and defective gaseous exchange causes all, except:

A. Prominent p wave
B. Decreased cerebral blood circulation
C. Increased red cell number
D. Pulmonary hypertension

18. Apnoea means:

A. Cessation of breathing
B. Shallow breathing
C. Distressed breathing
D. Increased breathing rate

19. What factor determines the quantity of gas that will diffuse through a barrier?

A. Molecular weight of diffusing particle
B. Solubility of particle in medium
C. Driving pressure
D. All of the above

20. Work done in quiet breathing is....... kg-m/breath.

A. 0.1 B. 0.2
C. 0.5 D. 2.5

21. During initial part of inspiration, which of the following does occur?

A. Intrapulmonary pressure falls
B. Intrathoracic pressure rises
C. Intra-abdominal pressure rises
D. The partial pressure of Oxygen in dead space rise

22. An increase in ventilation occurs in all except:

A. Fall in plasma bicarbonate
B. Sleep
C. Fall in pH of CSF
D. Rise in blood adrenaline level

23. The surfactant material lining the lung alveoli:

A. Decreases the surface tension of alveolar fluid
B. Increases the compliance of lungs

C. Has increasingly less effect, the more lungs are inflated
D. Is decreased when pulmonary blood flow is interrupted
E. All of the above

24. Contraction of smooth muscle in respiratory tract occurs in response to all, except:

A. Irritation of bronchial mucosa
B. Stimulation of local beta adrenoceptors
C. A decrease in the pCO_2 in the bronchial air
D. A cold stimulus to the bronchial mucosa

25. When the atmospheric pressure is halved, which of the following is not likely to develop?

A. An increase in pulmonary ventilation
B. A fall in arterial pO_2
C. A rise in arterial pH
D. A rise in cerebral blood flow

26. The Alveolar ventilation in an individual with Tidal volume: 600 ml, Dead space 150 ml and respiratory rate-15/min is........ L/min.

A. 2 B. 4.5
C. 6.75 D. 9

27. Normal value of FEV1 in an adult male is........%.

A. 95 B. 80
C. 65 D. 50

28. Spirometry measures all of the following except:

A. Tidal volume
B. Vital capacity
C. FEV1
D. None of the above

29. Surfactant is secreted by:

A. Pneumocyte I
B. Pneumocyte II
C. Goblet cells
D. Pulmonary vessels

30. FRC comprises:

A. Dead space volume
B. Residual volume
C. Volume of air present after normal expiration
D. Volume which can be inhaled after normal inspiration

31. The substance synthesized or stored in lung tissue and released into blood:

A. Histamine
B. Kallikrein
C. Prostaglandins E and F
D. All of the above

32. Respiratory minute volume in a normal person is .... L/min.

A. 1.2 B. 2
C. 4.2 D. 6

33. Max. mid exp. flow rate–indicates flow obstruction in:

A. Large airways
B. Small trachea
C. Trachea
D. Trachea and bronchi

34. Muscles of inspiration include which of the following?

A. Diaphragm and internal intercostals
B. Diaphragm and abdominal muscles
C. Abdominal muscles and external intercostals
D. Diaphragm and external intercostals

35. Consider the following statements:

Periodic (Cheyne-Stokes) breathing is seen:

1. After voluntary apnoea
2. After voluntary hyperpnoea
3. At high altitude
4. During wakeful states of adult human being

Of these statements:

A. 1 and 2 are correct
B. 1 and 3 are correct
C. 2,3 and 4 are correct
D. 1,3 and 4 are correct

36. In a normal adult, 24-hour production of CO_2 is about:

A. 150 L B. 280 L
C. 330 L D. 410 L

37. In a normal adult, the ratio of physiological and anatomical dead space is:

A. 2 :1 B. 1 :3
C. 3 :1 D. 1 :1

38. From lung to tissues O_2 transported is:

A. 70% B. 86%
C. 91% D. 97%

39. The renal body fluid volume mechanism for regulating arterial pressure is important for:

A. Raising the pressure when a person stands suddenly after having been in a lying position
B. Minimizing a decrease in arterial pressure following severe hemorrhage
C. Increasing arterial pressure during strenuous physical exercise
D. Maintaining arterial pressure at a normal level over a period of weeks, months or years

40. When CO_2 is removed in the lungs, which of the following also occur?

A. Efflux of HCO_3 from RBC
B. Efflux of Cl- from RBC
C. Efflux of CO_2
D. Efflux of O_2 and influx CO_2

41. Arterial pO_2 is reduced in:

A. Anaemia
B. KCN poisoning
C. Pulmonary hypoventilation
D. CO poisoning

42. What occurs in acclimatization to an high altitude?

A. Hyperventilation
B. Polycythemia
C. O_2 dissociation curve shifts to right
D. Decreased concentration of systemic capillaries

43. When CO_2 in inspired air increases beyond 10% at atmospheric pressure, it causes:

A. Decreased ventilation
B. Depression of CNS
C. Diminished sensory acuity
D. All of the above

44. An increase in ventilation occurs in all situations except:

A. Decrease plasma HCO_3^-
B. Sleep
C. Decreased pH in CSF
D. Increased blood adrenaline

45. The intrapleural pressure (mm Hg) at the end of deep inspiration is:

A. -4 B. +4
C. -18 D. +18

46. Total vital capacity is decreased but timed vital capacity is normal in:

A. Bronchial asthma
B. Scoliosis
C. Chronic bronchitis
D. All of the above

47. At a tidal volume of 500 ml, physiological dead space 150 ml and respiratory rate 12/min, the alveolar ventilation in ml/min is:

A. 6000 B. 4200
C. 180 D. 900

48. Circulation time through pulmonary capillaries is:

A. Less than 1 sec B. 10 sec
C. 20 sec D. 30 sec

49. Air in the pleural cavity causes all, except:

A. Reduction in residual volume
B. Abnormal dullness to percussion of the affected side
C. Less obvious rib contours on the affected side
D. Reduced vital capacity

50. As one ascends higher than 3000 m sea level, there is:

	PO_2	PCO_2
A.	Decrease	Increase
B.	Decrease	Decrease
C.	Increase	Increase
D.	Increase	Decrease

51. At 3000 m above sea level, PO_2 is about......mm Hg.

A. 70 B. 60
C. 50 D. 45

52. Oxygen toxicity limits exposures to less than......hours and pressures to.....atmospheres or less respectively.

A. 3,5 B. 5,3
C. 1 D. 2,1

53. Hyperbaric oxygenation is useful in all except:

A. Congenital heart disease
B. Gas gangrene
C. Carbon monoxide poisoning
D. Nitrogen toxicity

54. Cheyne-Stokes breathing is seen in:

A. CHF
B. Uremia
C. Brain
D. Any of the above

55. The ambient pressure increases by .... atmosphere for every 10 m of depth in sea water and every 10.4 of depth in fresh water.

A. 0.3 B. 0.8
C. 1.0 D. 1.8

56. Which is untrue about chloride shift?

A. Essentially complete in 1 sec
B. Chloride content of arterial blood is more than venous blood
C. Chloride content of arterial blood is less than venous blood
D. Diffusion of Cl- into the red cells

57. The respiratory minute volume is proportionate to the metabolic rate and the link between metabolism and ventilation is:

A. CO_2 B. O_2
C. Proteins D. All of the above

58. Carbon dioxide affects respiratory centre via:

A. Aortic bodies
B. Carotid bodies
C. Inflation and deflation receptors
D. CSF H^+ concentration

59. Stimuli affecting respiratory centre include:

A. CO_2 and O_2
B. Proprioceptors
C. Baroreceptors
D. All of the above

60. There is no stimulation of ventilation by hypoxia until the alveolar PO_2 falls below:

A. 60 mm Hg B. 58 mm Hg
C. 50 mm Hg D. 45 mm Hg

61. The stimulatory effects of hypoxia on ventilation do not clearly manifest until they become enough to override the counterbalancing inhibitory effects of a decline in:

A. Arterial H^+
B. Arterial H^+ and PCO_2
C. Venous H+
D. PO_2

62. The point at which breathing can no longer be voluntarily inhibited is called:

A. Herring Breuer reflex
B. Breaking point
C. Saturation point
D. Any of the above

63. During exercise, O_2 entering the blood may increase from 250 ml/min at rest to as high as......L/min.

A. 4 B. 10
C. 20 D. 30

64. In strenuous exercise, PO_2 (mm Hg) falls from:

A. 40 to 1 B. 60 to 35
C. 25 to 10 D. 35 to 0

65. The blood in the systemic arteries which bypass the pulmonary capillaries is about:

A. 0% B. 2%
C. 10% D. 15%

66. The following active substances are metabolized by the lung:

A. Kallikrien
B. Serotonin
C. Angiotensin I-Angiotensin II
D. All of the above

67. Timed vital capacity in 3 sec is:

A. 83% B. 87%
C. 97% D. 99.9%

68. Tidal volume in both men and women is:

A. 250 ml B. 500 ml
C. 1000 ml D. 1200 ml

69. The total area of the alveolar walls in contact with capillaries in both lungs is about ......sq. m.

A. 10 B. 30
C. 70 D. 120

70. There are about......million alveoli in man.

A. 50 B. 100
C. 300 D. 500

71. Vital capacity in men is:

A. 4.2 L B. 4.8 L
C. 6.0 L D. 6.8 L

72. Which of the following volume is equal in both men and women?

A. Inspiratory reserve volume
B. Tidal volume
C. Residual volume
D. Vital capacity

EXPLANATORY ANSWERS OF RESPIRATION

1. **Ans. B:** Alveolar ventilation is the amount of air ventilating the alveoli per minute.

   Alveolar ventilation = (Tidal volume – Dead space) × Respiratory rate

   = (500-150) × 12

   = 4200 ml. (AK Jain 449)

2. **Ans. C:** Respiratory distress syndrome is a serious disease of new born infants, due to deficiency of surfactant. It develops in infants who are preterm, i.e., they are born before their surfactant becomes functional. (AK Jain 442)

3. **Ans. A:** CO_2 enter into capillaries by diffusion. Arterial blood pCO_2 is 40 mm Hg. Tissue pCO_2 is 46 mm Hg. Diffusion occurs from Tissue to blood due to difference in pCO_2. (AK Jain 461)

4. **Ans. A:** Affinity of carbonmonoxide to combine with haemoglobin is 200 times more than that of oxygen. Higher affinity of CO for haemoglobin produces large proportions of haemoglobin (CO-Hb) and therefore, haemoglobin is unavailable for oxygen carriage. CO shifts the oxygen dissociation curve to the left due to inhibition of synthesis of 2,3 DPG. (AK Jain 57, 458)

5. **Ans. A:** Work of breathing is 0.3 to 0.8 kgmt/min. Elastic resistance is 65%. Non elastic resistance (1) Viscous 7% (2) Airway resistance 28%. Most of the energy is spent in overcoming elastic resistance. (AK Jain 448)

6. **Ans. D:** Chemical stimuli like CO_2, O_2 and H+ affect respiratory centre. (AK Jain 470)

7. **Ans. B:** Average = 100 l/min. It is the largest volume of air that can be moved into and out of the lung in one minute by maximum voluntary effort. (AK Jain 440)

8. **Ans. D:** Increase in HCO_3^- concentration occurs in hypoventilation, Decrease in HCO_3^- concentration occurs in Hyperventilation. Acidosis (decrease in HCO_3^- and increase in H+ concentration) increases respiration. Alkalosis (increase in HCO_3^- and decrease in H+ concentration) result in hypoventilation. These effects are mediated via peripheral chemoreceptor. (AK Jain 498) In small doses, adrenaline stimulates respiration by stimulation of peripheral chemoreceptors. In high doses, it raises the systemic arterial blood pressure, which inhibits the respiration producing apnoea, called Adrenaline apnoea. (AK Jain 472)

9. **Ans. D:** Pulmonary ventilation is the amount of air ventilating the alveoli per minute. Pulmonary ventilation = (Tidal volume – Dead space) × Respiratory rate. Dead space is the volume of air in the respiratory passage which does not take part in exchange of gases (wasted pulmonary ventilation). However if the patient's pulmonary ventilation is greater than the respiratory rate, it means that he is respiring in dead space. Dead space increases in emphysema, bronchiectasis and pulmonary embolism. It remains constant in rapid shallow respiration and slow and deep respiration, i.e., 150 ml. (AK Jain 424)

10. **Ans. B:** In high altitude, decrease arterial PO_2 stimulates peripheral chemoreceptor and increases pulmonary ventilation, CO_2 wash out, decreasing alveolar pCO_2 that decreases H+ concentration in blood (alkalosis) and this should inhibit respiration. (AK Jain 497)

11. **Ans. B:** The chemical regulatory mechanism adjust ventilation in such a way that the alveolar pCO_2 is kept constant at normal value of 40 mm Hg. (AK Jain 473)
12. **Ans. C:** Tidal volume is 500 ml. Volume of air breathed in or out of lung during quiet breathing. (AK Jain 435)
13. **Ans. A:** Inspiratory reserve volume is 2000 to 3200 ml. The maximum volume of air which can be inspired after completing a normal tidal inspiration, i.e., inspiration from the end inspiratory position. (AK Jain 435)
14. **Ans. B:** Vital capacity is 4.8 L in males and 3.2 L in females. It is the maximal amount of air that can be expelled from the lungs by forceful effort following a maximum inspiration. (AK Jain 435)
15. **Ans. D:** Inspiratory capacity is the maximal volume of air which can be inspired after completing tidal expiration. Vital capacity is 2500 to 3700 ml. (AK Jain 435)
16. **Ans. A:** CO_2 has high diffusion coefficient of about 20 times more than that of O_2. (AK Jain 461)
17. **Ans. B:** Cerebral blood flow is well regulated at arterial pressure of 65-140 mm Hg and shows no change. Defective gas exchange causes hypoxia that causes marked increase in pulmonary arterial pressure or pulmonary hypertension, that leads to right atrial hypertrophy (prominent p wave), right ventricular hypertrophy, right heart failure and pulmonary oedema. Hypoxia also stimulates erythropoiesis resulting in increased red cell membrane. (Ganong 610)
18. **Ans. A:** Apnoea means stoppage of all respiration. (AK Jain 468)
19. **Ans. D:** Factors that affect rate of diffusion:
$$D \propto \frac{\Delta P \times SA \times SOL}{T \times \sqrt{MW}}$$
Where D is the quantity of gas that diffuses through a barrier in given time

    MW is molecular weight of substance

    SOL is solubility of particle in medium

    Δ P is the driving pressure

    SA is the surface area

    T is the temperature

    The molecules of each species diffuse independently. (AK Jain 12,14)
20. **Ans. C:** Work of breathing is 0.3 to 0.8 kgmt/min. Elastic resistance is 65%. Non-elastic resistance (1) Viscous 7% (2) Airway resistance 28%. Most of the energy is used in overcoming elastic resistance. (AK Jain 448)
21. **Ans. B:** The intrapulmonary pressure decreases due to expansion of lung. At the end of expiratory position, the tendency of the lung to recoil from the chest wall is just balanced by tendency of chest wall to move in the opposite direction. This causes slight subatmospheric pressure to develop, i.e., -2 mm of Hg between two layers of pleura at start of inspiration. (AK Jain 433)
22. **Ans. B:** The sensitivity of CO_2 on respiration decreased by sleep, anesthesia and hypothermia. It is increased by hypoxia, hyperthermia. (AK Jain 480)
23. **Ans. E:** Surfactant decreases surface tension. When lungs are inflated in inspiration it is less effective. Surfactant decreases due to occlusion of one pulmonary artery. (AK Jain 441, 442)
24. **Ans. B:** Stimulation of adrenoreceptor produces smooth muscle relaxation. Asthma or bronchoconstriction is worsened in the cold. (AK Jain 955)
25. **Ans. D:** Arterial pO_2 decreases it stimulates peripheral chemoreceptors to increase respiration. Hyperventilation increases CO_2 washout, decreasing alveolar pCO_2

and decreases H+ concentration in blood (alkalosis). This inhibits respiration. As a result in acclimatized state ventilation shows no change. Cerebral blood flow is well regulated at arterial pressure of 65-140 mm Hg and shows no change. (AK Jain 497, Ganong 610)

26. **Ans. C:** Alveolar ventilation = (Tidal volume – Dead space) × Respiratory rate

    = (600-150) × 15

    = 6750 ml. (AK Jain 449)

27. **Ans. B:** Forced vital capacity FVC is the maximum volume of air that can be breathed out as forcefully and rapidly as possible following a maximum inspiration. FEV1 or forced Expiratory Volume in One second of exhalation is 80% of FVC. FEV2 in two seconds is 95%. FEV3 in first three seconds of exhalation is 98-100%. (AK Jain 438)

28. **Ans. D:** With the exception of FRC, all other lung volume and capacities can be measured with the help of simple spirometer. (AK Jain 437)

29. **Ans. B:** Surfactant is secreted by granular pneumocyte, i.e., Alveolar lining epithelium. Type II cells and comes to the surface by exocytosis. It is removed by pulmonary alveolar macrophages. (AK Jain 440)

30. **Ans. C:** Functional residual capacity is volume of air which is contained in lungs at end expiratory position. Normal is 2.5 litres. It acts as a buffer allowing continuous exchange of gases to occur even during expiration thereby prevents sudden changes in partial pressure of gases in blood. (AK Jain 437)

31. **Ans. D:** Substance synthesized or stored and released into blood are: Prostaglandin, Histamine, Kallikrien. (AK Jain 430)

32. **Ans. B:** Alveolar ventilation = (Tidal volume – Dead space) × Respiratory rate

    = (500-150) × 12

    = 4200 ml. (AK Jain 449)

33. **Ans. B:** Peak expiratory flow rate is the maximum flow of air achieved during measurement of forced vital capacity. It is an index of mid sized airway function. Maximum Mid Expiratory Flow Rate (MMEFR) is the mean expiratory flow rate during 50% of FVC. Normal is 300 L/min. (AK Jain 440, 502-503)

34. **Ans. D:** Diaphragm is the main muscle of inspiration. The external intercostals muscles supplied by T_1, T_2 cause an increase in anterior-posterior diameter of ribs (second to sixth) as they move outwards in inspiration (Pump handle movement). The lower ribs (7th and 10th) also swing outward and upwards in inspiration to cause an increase of transverse diameter (Bucket handle movement). (AK Jain 431)

35. **Ans. A:** Cheyne-Stokes respiration is a periodic form of breathing that is caused by (A) Physiological (a) Voluntary Hyperventilation (b) High altitude (c) During sleep in some normal individuals (B) Pathological (a) Heart failure (b) Brain damage (c) Uremia. (AK Jain 482)

36. **Ans. B:** 280 L CO_2 produced in 24 hours. 4 ml% is transported in blood. Out of which 0.3% is in dissolved form, 0.7 ml% is in carbamino compounds and 3 ml% as bicarbonate. (AK Jain 461)

37. **Ans. D:** Physiologic and anatomic dead space is not same in pathological conditions because of closed capillaries or poorly perfused lungs. It is same in a normal individual. (AK Jain 449-451)

38. **Ans. D:** 97% is Hb-O_2 saturation, rest is dissolved in plasma. (AK Jain 456)

39. **Ans. D:** Renal body fluid volume for regulating arterial pressure is a long-term over period of weeks, months. This includes rennin angiotensin system. Choice A is the

baroreceptor mechanism for beat to beat regulation every second. (AK Jain 346)

40. **Ans. B:** Carbon dioxide washout, HCO_3- is exchanged with Cl- that moves out of the RBC. This is opposite to chloride shift in venous blood, where the packed cell volume is more than arterial blood. The cells are larger because of influx of Chloride brings water along. (AK Jain 464)
41. **Ans. C:** In anemic hypoxia and Carbon-monoxide poisoning despite the normal arterial pO_2 decreased amount of hemoglobin causes decreased tissue oxygen. KCN and are examples of histotoxic hypoxia. Here again normal arterial pO_2 is there but due to the toxic agent the tissue cannot utilize oxygen. In pulmonary hypoventilation however decreased arterial pO_2 is present, normal oxygen carrying capacity and rate of blood flow to the tissues exist. (AK Jain 490)
42. **Ans. C:** High altitude acclimatization changes occur at three levels: lungs, blood, tissues. Ascent to high altitude triggers a substantial rise in 2,3 DPG concentration in RBC, shifting the oxygen dissociation curve to right. The systemic capillaries open at tissues. Polycythemia and Hyperventilation does not occur once the person has acclimatized to the high altitude. (AK Jain 497)
43. **Ans. D:** Increase in carbon dioxide > 7% causes CNS depression, reducing ventilation and threshold of reticular formation. This is called carbon dioxide narcosis. (AK Jain 477)
44. **Ans. B:** In sleep the energy rests in the spine, away from the lungs. The breath slows, the body rests. Stimulants of respiration are adrenaline in exercise to give more oxygen to lungs, H^+ ions (decreased pH). HCO_3^- has no direct role, though its value is important to diagnose conditions of respiratory acidosis. (AK Jain 472)
45. **Ans. A:** The negative intrapleural pressure is directly proportional to amount of thoracic expansion. Intrapleural pressure is the pressure between the visceral and parietal pleura (the coverings of the lungs). In inspiration this pressure is negative to the atmosphere, to enable air to move in the lungs. At the end of deep inspiration it is -6 mm of Hg. -4 mm of Hg is the closest choice. (AK Jain 430)
46. **Ans. B:** Timed vital capacity is the maximum volume of air which can be breathed out as forcefully and rapidly as possible following a maximum inspiration. Scoliosis is a restrictive disease (also kyphoscoliosis, ankylosing spondylitis), in which the back is bent sidewards, chest expansion is resticted. Lungs is like a tank whose opening is the bronchus. In fibrosis also the volume of lung, i.e., its capacity decreases but FEV1 is normal. In obstructive the opening is decreased in size. So the rate of flow of air (timed vital capacity) through the narrow opening is less in bronchial asthma, chronic bronchitis, emphysema (Obstructive diseases), i.e., VC is normal but FEV1 decreases. (AK Jain 438)
47. **Ans. B:** Alveolar ventilation = (Tidal volume – Dead space) × Respiratory rate
    = (500-150) × 12
    = 4200 ml. (AK Jain 449)
48. **Ans. A:** Pulmonary capillaries are 4 µm in radius and 350 µm long. A network of pulmonary capillaries surrounds the alveoli and is sandwiched between their walls. At rest: Effective surface wall surface area increases to 60 m^2 and transit time is one second. During heavy exercise area increases to 90 m^2 and transit time to 0.3 seconds. (AK Jain 405)
49. **Ans. B:** Air in pleural cavity causes collapse of lung due to equalization of intrapleural pressure with atmospheric pressure. This decreases the vital capacity and residual

volume. Due to air there is increased resonance on percussion. (AK Jain 435)

50. **Ans. B:** A height in excess of 10,000 feet (3000 m) above sea level is defined as high altitude. Hyperpnoea (increase in breathing) occurs at high altitude when arterial pO_2 falls below 60 mm Hg, resulting in fall in alveolar pCO_2. (AK Jain 494)
51. **Ans. B:** A height in excess of 10,000 feet (3000 m) above sea level is defined as high altitude. Hyperpnoea (increase in breathing) occurs at high altitude when arterial pO_2 falls below 60 mm Hg, resulting in fall in alveolar pCO_2. (AK Jain 494)
52. **Ans. B:** Administration of 80-100% O_2 for more than 8 hours will stimulate irritant receptors. For more than 24 hours will cause bronchopneumonia. At "three" atmospheric pressure, inhalation of 100% causes oxygen toxicity quite early. (AK Jain 492)
53. **Ans. D:** Inhalation of 100% oxygen at high barometric pressure is called hyperbaric oxygen therapy. Inhalation of 100% oxygen at one atmospheric pressure is useful in hypoxic hypoxia. It has limited value in anaemic, stagnant and histotoxic hypoxia. Nitrogen toxicity causes High pressure nervous syndrome that is treated by compressing and slowly decompressing to dissolve the nitrogen bubbles and release it. Oxygen Helium mixture are used instead of nitrogen. (AK Jain 491, 501)
54. **Ans. D:** Cheyne-Stokes respiration is a periodic form of breathing that is caused by (A) Physiological (a) Voluntary Hyperventilation (b) High altitude (c) During sleep in some normal individuals (B) Pathological (a) Heart failure (b) Brain damage (c) Uremia. (AK Jain 482)
55. **Ans. C:** For every 33 feet (10 meters) deep down in sea there will occur an increase in pressure by one atmospheric pressure. In fresh water it is for every 10.4 meters. (AK Jain 500)
56. **Ans. C:** Carbon dioxide accumulation in venous blood, HCO_3- removed from the RBC. Cl- moves into of the cell. This is chloride shift. Thus in venous blood, the packed cell volume is more than arterial blood. The cells are larger because of influx of Chloride brings water along. (AK Jain 464)
57. **Ans. A:** Alveolar pCO_2 depends upon balance between metabolism of body and respiration. When body metabolism increases, alveolar pCO_2 increases, CO_2 is washed out, restoring alveolar pCO_2. Opposite is seen when body metabolism decreases. (AK Jain 494)
58. **Ans. D:** Medullary (central) chemoreceptors are located on the ventral surface of medulla near the respiratory centre. They get stimulated by the H+ concentration of CSF. The magnitude of stimulation is directly proportional to local increase in H+ concentration, which increases in linearity with the arterial pCO_2. These chemoreceptor get inhibited by anaesthesia, cyanide and during sleep. (AK Jain 497, 498)
59. **Ans. D:** Factors affecting respiratory centre (a) Chemical stimulation: CO_2 ,O_2 and H + (b) Non-chemical stimuli (i) Afferent from higher centre (ii) Vagal afferent from inhalation and deflation receptors in the lungs (iii) Afferent from proprioceptors (iv) Afferent from pharynx, trachea and bronchi (v) Afferent from baroreceptor (vi) Chemoreceptors (carotid and aortic bodies). (AK Jain 470, 471)
60. **Ans. A:** A height in excess of 10,000 feet (3000 m) above sea level is defined as high altitude. Hyperpnoea (increase in breathing) occurs at high altitude when arterial pO_2 falls below 60 mm Hg, resulting in fall in alveolar pCO_2. (AK Jain 494)
61. **Ans. B:** In high altitude, decrease arterial pO_2 stimulates peripheral chemoreceptor and *increases* pulmonary ventilation, CO_2 wash out, decreasing alveolar pCO_2 that decreases H+ concentration in blood

(alkalosis) and this should *inhibit* respiration. (AK Jain 497)

62. **Ans. B:** Breath-holding occurs for a period of 45-55 seconds in normal healthy subjects. The point at which breathing can no longer be voluntary inhibited is called Breaking point. It is due to increased arterial pCO_2 and decreased arterial pO_2. (AK Jain 481)

63. **Ans. A:** During exercise VO_2 (oxygen consumption) increases 15-20 times from the resting value of 250 ml/min due to increase in cardiac output, increase alveolar ventilation, capillary density and RBC count. (AK Jain 508)

64. **Ans. A:** Strenuous exercise is defined as that in which heart rate increases to 150/min and oxygen consumption is 75% of resting value. In this pulmonary ventilation increases disproportionately due to anaerobiosis of the working muscles, which contributes an extra drive to working muscles, which contributes an extra drive to respiratory centre. Even at low pO_2 the tissues can utilize oxygen as oxygen dissociation curve shifts to the right due to rise in temperature, increase in arterial pCO_2, decrease arterial pO_2 and decrease in arterial pH. (AK Jain 508)

65. **Ans. B:** Bronchopulmonary circulation accounts for about 2% of systemic circulation. These supply the bronchus and lungs. (AK Jain 404, 429)

66. **Ans. D:** Substance metabolized are serotonin, prostaglandin, bradykinin, adenine derivative, acetylcholine, nor epinephrine. (AK Jain 430)

67. **Ans. C:** Forced vital capacity FVC is the maximum volume of air that can be breathed out as forcefully and rapidly as possible following a maximum inspiration. FEV1 or forced Expiratory Volume in One second of exhalation is 80% of FVC. FEV2 in two seconds is 95%. FEV3 in first three seconds of exhalation is 98-100%. (AK Jain 438)

68. **Ans. B:** Tidal volume is 500 ml. Volume of air breathed in or out of lung during quiet breathing. (AK Jain 435)

69. **Ans. C:** Surface area > 70 m^2. (AK Jain 424)

70. **Ans. C:** 300 million alveoli are there in the two lungs. Surface area > 70 m^2. (AK Jain 424)

71. **Ans. B:** Vital capacity in men is 4.8 litre. This maximal volume of air is expelled from the lungs by forceful effort following a maximal inspiration. (AK Jain 436)

72. **Ans. B:** Tidal volume is 500 ml. Volume of air breathed in or out of lung during quiet breathing. (AK Jain 435)